Exercise Physiology - Bridging Health, Training Performance and Technology

Edited by Samuel Honório

Published in London, United Kingdom

Exercise Physiology - Bridging Health, Training Performance and Technology
http://dx.doi.org/10.5772/intechopen.1008596
Edited by Samuel Honório

Contributors
Bernelee Denize Doherty, Chaoyang Wang, Dimitar Avramov, Ensley Tanner, Hannah Griffin, Kai Liu, Kuang-Drew Li, Meha Fatima Aftab, Mukoma G. Gudani, Musa L. Mathunjwa, Rajavi Solanki, Rohan Sharma, Senzelwe Mazibuko, Soham Kulkarni, Tathya Patel, Terry Jeremy Ellapen, Thomas Hornaday, Vincent J.B. Robinson, Xiaodong Zhang, Yahui Zhang, Zsolt Bagi

First published in London, United Kingdom, 2026 by IntechOpen
IntechOpen is the global imprint of INTECHOPEN LIMITED, registered in England and Wales, registration number: 11086078, 167-169 Great Portland Street, London, W1W 5PF, United Kingdom

For EU product safety concerns: IN TECH d.o.o., Prolaz Marije Krucifikse Kozulić 3, 51000 Rijeka, Croatia, info@intechopen.com or visit our website at intechopen.com.

British Library Cataloguing-in-Publication Data
A catalogue record for this book is available from the British Library

Exercise Physiology - Bridging Health, Training Performance and Technology
Edited by Samuel Honório
p. cm.
Print ISBN 978-1-83635-617-2
Online ISBN 978-1-83635-616-5
eBook (PDF) ISBN 978-1-83635-618-9

Meet the editor

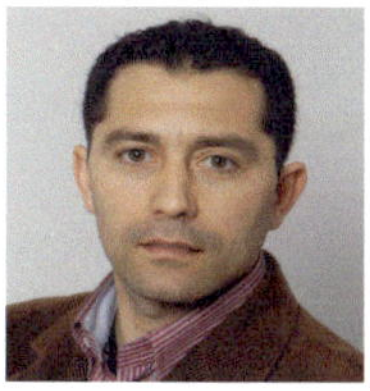

Dr. Samuel Honório is a full-time teacher at the Polytechnic Institute of Castelo Branco, Portugal. He is a member of the Sports Science and Well-Being Department. Serves as an Adjunct Professor, has a Ph.D. in Sport Sciences and a Post-doctorate graduation in Physical Activity and Health, with several investigations in the field of Healthy Habits and Lifestyles, physiology, and motor competence. He also has a Master's degree in Education Sciences and a bachelor's degree in teaching of Physical Activity. He is also an author and co-author of several books and articles in the field. It believes in the educational and formative value of sport, in a much broader dimension than simply regular physical activity, across several domains of modern society. It is dedicated to a core set of elements that serve as fundamental indicators of scientific rigor and professional ethics.

Contents

Preface

The evolution and transformation within sports sciences have changed the way we understand human body function, physical performance, and the mechanisms that support it in the field of health and performance. Exercise physiology is now integrating clinical and technological practices, establishing an increasingly solid connection between scientific knowledge, effort monitoring, and ways to optimize human performance.

This work, *Exercise Physiology – Bridging Health, Training Performance and Technology*, arises from the need to integrate diverse areas of knowledge into a modern, interdisciplinary vision. Exercise physiology provides the basis for understanding the body's responses and adaptations to physical exertion, with performance reflecting these adaptations across different contexts. Technology emerges as a mediating and enhancing element, enabling more precise measurement of interventions and decision-making.

Currently, technological tools such as sensors, devices, monitoring software, and digital platforms have revolutionized the way health professionals and trainers interpret the signals of the human body. This integration not only improves physical performance but also promotes safety, injury prevention, individualized training, and more efficient strategies for cardiovascular rehabilitation and health promotion. This work proposes a reflection on the convergence between science, practice, and technological innovation, highlighting how physiological understanding can be broadened through modern methods of functional analysis and monitoring. More than presenting isolated concepts, this work seeks to build an integrated vision in which physiology, performance, and technology coexist in a complementary and strategic way.

In these chapters, the reader will find discussions based on scientific evidence on cardiovascular and metabolic adaptations to exercise and on technological applications in functional assessment. The goal is to contribute to an update of content for students, researchers, and professionals interested in understanding how the union between exercise physiology, performance, and technology works.

This book is intended to serve as a point of connection between scientific knowledge and practical application, inspiring new investigations, new methodologies, and new ways of understanding human potential through movement.

Samuel Honório
Department of Sport Sciences and Well-being,
Polytechnic University of Castelo Branco,
Castelo Branco, Portugal

Section 1

Cardiovascular Adaptations in Exercise

Chapter 1

Cardiac Output Enhancement: New Insights into the Mechanisms That Engage Diastolic Function Optimization during Aerobic Exercise

Vincent J.B. Robinson, Soham Kulkarni, Rohan Sharma, Thomas Hornaday, Ensley Tanner, Kuang-Drew Li, Tathya Patel, Rajavi Solanki, Hannah Griffin and Zsolt Bagi

Abstract

Aerobic exercise elicits profound cardiovascular adaptations focused on maximizing diastolic function, which enables the heart to meet the increased circulatory demands imposed by physical exertion. This chapter explores how the low-pressure compartments contribute to improving cardiac output through optimized diastolic filling. Central to these adaptations are structural and functional changes in venous conduit vessels, such as the inferior vena cava (IVC) and the pulmonary vasculature. Aerobic exercise-induced IVC remodeling, blood volume mobilization, and pulmonary transit time reduction all facilitate preload augmentation without significant increases in venous resistance. At the myocardial level, cardiac auxotonic relaxation supports early diastolic filling during shortened diastolic phases, aided by physiological left ventricular eccentric hypertrophy and coronary vascular expansion, which leads to metabolic balance between substrate supply and energy production. Another critical mediator of the processes enhancing diastolic function is adenosine, which not only promotes vasodilation in conduit and coronary vessels but also supports auxotonic relaxation and capillary angiogenesis. Together, these integrated adaptations in the venous, pulmonary, myocardial, and coronary systems underscore the critical role of diastolic enhancement in sustaining high cardiac output during aerobic performance. This chapter offers a comprehensive review of the structural and functional mechanisms underlying these processes and highlights the underappreciated but essential contributions of the low-pressure compartment in enhancing diastolic function and achieving maximal aerobic exercise capacity.

Keywords: auxotonic relaxation, adenosine, venous resistance, lusiotropy, E/A ratio, E/e′ ratio, eccentric hypertrophy, pulmonary transit time, blood volume reservoir, low-pressure compartment, metabolic vasoregulation, endurance training

1. Introduction

Exercise plays a vital role in maintaining physical and mental health. Whether it be an intense gym workout session or a brisk walk around the neighborhood, regular physical activity has been shown to improve overall wellbeing. It is a modifiable risk factor for cardiovascular disease, including diabetes, hypertension, and obesity [1]. The link between physical activity and cardiovascular disease became widely recognized in the medical field back in 1996, when the American Heart Association (AHA) released findings highlighting the positive impact of exercise on hemodynamic, hormonal, metabolic, neurological, and respiratory functions for the first time [2]. Engaging in physical activity has been associated with lower risk of death from any cause in older adults [3]. People who tend to exercise regularly live longer, healthier, and more active lives.

Physical activity is broadly classified into two basic categories of aerobic and isometric form, each offering distinct benefits for health and fitness. The American College of Sports Medicine describes aerobic exercise as a rhythmic activity involving large muscle groups that can be performed continuously over time. Aerobic exercise can vary from light to vigorous levels of intensity. Aerobic activities improve cardiovascular endurance by facilitating positive adaptive changes in the heart and lungs, which enhances cardiac output and leads to a sustained increase in oxygen delivery throughout the body. According to the CDC National Center for Health Statistics, 46.9% of adults age 18 or above meet the Physical Activity Guidelines for daily aerobic exercise [4]. Studies have shown that aerobic exercise helps reduce blood pressure, lower cholesterol/triglycerides, enhance insulin sensitivity, and positively impact all dimensions of cardiovascular health [2, 5].

The cardiovascular system is a primary driver of the physiological changes occurring during exercise. As one of the oldest and most extensively studied fields in medicine, cardiovascular physiology has laid the foundation for understanding human aerobic exercise and performance. William Harvey, a seventeenth-century physician, in his 1628 publication "Exercitatio anatomica de motu cordis et sanguinis in animalibus" (on the motion of the heart and blood in animals) was the first to correctly distinguish between the presumed passive filling of the heart (diastole) and its active pumping mechanism (systole), which laid the foundation for understanding the separate physiologic demands of systole and diastole [6]. Physiologist Otto Frank and anatomist Ernest Starling introduced the revolutionary Frank-Starling curve in 1899, characterizing the positive relation between stroke volume and end-diastolic volume.

Maintaining end-diastolic volume during the shortened diastolic filling time of aerobic exercise can prove to be a physiologic challenge. The low-pressure compartments of the circulatory system play a pivotal role in supporting and enhancing diastolic function during aerobic exercise. These primarily refer to regions of the circulatory system where blood is transported and stored under relatively low hydrostatic pressure. During aerobic exercise, the systemic venous system and pulmonary vasculature, essential components of the low-pressure circuit, become increasingly important in enhancing preload and augmenting cardiac output [7]. This is facilitated by structural remodeling and dilation of a major venous return conduit (the inferior vena cava (IVC)), sympathetic activated mobilization of blood volume, and decreased pulmonary transit associated with capillary recruitment and improved gas exchange. Together, these adaptations optimize diastolic filling to meet the elevated circulatory demands of aerobic exercise.

Guyton and colleagues investigated how epinephrine increases cardiac output, with a particular focus on its effect on venous return [8]. Although the concept of diastolic function was not fully understood at the time, their work laid the foundational framework for recognizing the role of diastolic filling in governing cardiac output, which can be applied to dynamic conditions such as aerobic exercise. In his classic 1958 study of mobilizing venous capacitance to increase cardiac output in denervated dogs, Guyton showed that as cardiac output increased, there was no increase in venous resistance. As venous resistance is determined by the biomechanical determinants of laminar flow, for it to remain constant in the presence of increasing flow, there must be venous conduit dilation, which Guyton did not explicitly observe. In this chapter, we plan to show agents that promote IVC conduit vein dilation are linked to increases in cardiac output, hence the ability to lower/stabilize venous resistance in times of increased venous return.

Aerobic exercise presents a particular challenge to diastolic filling: cardiac output typically ranges from 5 to 6 L/min at rest but exceeds 35 L/min in elite athletes during intense activity [9]. How does the heart accommodate a sevenfold increase in blood flow when diastolic filling time is reduced to about one-fifth of its resting duration? The answer lies in exponential enhancement of diastolic function through major anatomic and physiologic adaptations; otherwise, aerobic exercise would not be possible. To meet the increased circulatory demands, the cardiovascular system employs multiple mechanisms to optimize diastolic filling. Unlike skeletal muscle, cardiac muscle undergoes auxotonic relaxation where both pressure and volume (or length) change at the same time in the ventricle during relaxation [10]. This allows the increased central translocation of blood from the lusitropic adaptations within the low-pressure compartment to fill the ventricles more rapidly and at lower filling pressures. Details of the adaptations that make this possible will be reviewed later in this chapter.

With prolonged and intense physical training, the heart itself undergoes significant structural adaptations to meet the increased demands of exercise. By the late nineteenth century, cardiac enlargement in athletes had already been observed, initially detected through chest percussion in cross-country skiers, was later validated through radiographic imaging [11]. Swedish physician Salomon Henschen first described the term "athlete's heart" back in 1899 through his observation of cardiac enlargement and hypertrophy in cross-country skiers [12]. Athlete's heart is characterized by physiological left ventricular enlargement and mild myocardial hypertrophy, which enhance diastolic function by increasing ventricular end diastolic volume. These adaptations, which increase cardiac end diastolic volume, enable the heart to sustain high cardiac output during intense physical activity without requiring excessive increases in heart rate.

When functioning at peak metabolic capacity, the cardiac pump requires increases in substrate levels to maintain its systolic and diastolic performance. Adenosine is suggested as the biochemical modulator of cardiac energetics and blood flow. In this context, early studies, notably those by Drury, Szent-Gyorgyi and Berne, identified adenosine as a key metabolic signal that links increased ATP turnover to local vasodilation and myocardial adaptation during maximal exercise [13, 14]. As ATP is rapidly broken-down during exercise, adenosine builds up and activates receptor-mediated pathways that enhance coronary blood flow and myocardial relaxation, critical processes for maintaining cardiac output. These actions are essential for preserving diastolic efficiency and contractile performance under higher workload conditions. Simultaneously, adenosine helps regulate blood flow in systemic low-pressure areas, contributing to metabolic flow control across various organ systems. The important role of adenosine in coordinating heart and vessel responses to increased metabolic needs will be discussed in detail in the final part of this chapter, focusing on adenosine receptor-specific mechanisms and their physiological significance.

While most research has traditionally focused on systolic performance during exercise, the mechanisms that enhance diastolic filling, particularly the roles of the pulmonary circulation and the systemic low-pressure venous conduit and reservoir, remain underappreciated and poorly understood. In this chapter, we aim to fill this gap in knowledge with a view of integrated changes within the low-pressure and cardiac compartments. Experimental literature is sparse, but we use conceptual studies to present an integrated hypothesis to hopefully stimulate new experimental studies in this area. We examine how adaptations in the low-pressure compartments of the cardiovascular system, including pulmonary vascular and conduit vein remodeling, cardiac auxotonic relaxation, and adenosine work in concert to optimize diastolic filling and overall cardiac efficiency. These adaptations are accompanied by vascular remodeling that can be applied to improving diastolic function in other chronic disease states.

2. Low pressure compartment adaptations facilitating diastolic function in aerobic exercise

2.1 Venous capacitance, compliance, and total blood volume

The performance of aerobic exercise relies on one's ability to enhance diastolic filling. In this section, we focus on the adaptations of the systemic venous system to translocate blood into the cardiac and pulmonary reservoirs. Crucial for enhanced filling are adaptations in venous return that facilitate increase in cardiac output. The low-pressure compartment, from venules to larger conduit veins, is mainly responsible for left and right ventricular loading. This system holds approximately 80% of blood volume, leaving 20% to be held within the higher-pressure systems. This distribution of blood is unstressed and exerts no transmural pressure on venous walls [15]. However, when considering venous flow and its impact on cardiac output, unstressed volume must be recruited as stressed volume in order to influence mean systemic pressure and venous return. Stressed volume, accounting for approximately 30% of total blood volume, is the amount of blood exerting pressure within the venous system. Both unstressed and stressed volumes make up vascular capacitance, which is the ability of blood vessels to hold volume within a specific region of the cardiovascular system. When catecholamine surges occur, venous capacitance is mobilized to load the central compartment. As stressed volume increases, it appears that conduit veins may dilate due to their reduced sympathetic innervation and relatively increased compliance [16].

2.2 Blood volume shifts and reservoir creation with upright exercise

Because cardiac output is the product of stroke volume and heart rate, blood volume filling the heart during diastole must increase to accommodate cardiac output during exercise. The Frank Starling Law further implies that increased end diastolic volume contributes to increased stroke volume leading to enhanced cardiac output. It is evidenced that splanchnic capacitance plays a role in hemodynamic stability by acting as a reservoir. The splanchnic blood reservoir has demonstrated its compliance capability in multiple settings including hemorrhage, splanchnic nerve stimulation, and responses to epinephrine. This splanchnic response is elicited in cats after loading and depleting blood volume. The splanchnic beds were able to sequester or pool 50–70% of blood volume as a result of adding or depleting volume [17]. During exercise, there is a consensus that the splanchnic reservoir decreases in volume [18–20].

In a landmark study, Flamm et al. studied whole body images that utilized gamma camera detecting technetium 99 m labeled red blood cells. Their work revealed that with increased aerobic exercise during upright cycling in healthy individuals, abdominal and lower extremity blood volume decreased while thoracic blood volume increased. Notably, blood volume in the spleen decreased by 46%, followed by the kidney and liver at 24% and 18%, respectively. Meanwhile, the blood volume of the thoracic cavity increased by 38% [21]. This suggests that as one exercises, blood volume from the splanchnic reservoir contributes to the creation of a thoracic reservoir of blood to fill the left ventricle (LV) in times of rapidly increasing LV filling.

Musch et al. describe a similar phenomenon. However, their exercise study was performed in dogs [22]. Both Flamm et al. and Musch et al.'s studies demonstrate that exercise induces a marked redistribution of blood volume to support the increased cardiac output required by working skeletal muscle. These shifts in blood volume appear to be linked to dramatic changes in splanchnic and renal blood flow which decrease substantially during exercise, with values falling from approximately 3 liters per minute at rest to less than 1 liter per minute, thereby reallocating up to 2 liters per minute of cardiac output to active muscle tissue [23]. Braunwald et al. also describe an increase in central (thoracic) blood volume in healthy, exercising adult males accompanied by increased cardiac output [24]. However, the study by Flamm et al. uniquely characterizes both the source and destination of this mobilized blood, demonstrating that the thoracic cavity serves as a reservoir for the redistributed splanchnic blood volume during exercise. This study serves as a clear indication that the splanchnic reservoir plays a role in maintaining blood volume and cardiac output requirements during aerobic exercise by mobilizing volume for enhanced preload. Similarly, the study by Flamm et al. shows that when heart rate increases, the filling time decreases by a proportional amount. As filling time shortened, end diastolic volume remained stable, suggesting increasingly effective blood mobilization and LV filling throughout the duration of aerobic exercise.

2.3 IVC remodeling in aerobic trained athletes

As discussed above, an increase in blood volume in the thoracic vessels is accomplished through mobilization from the splanchnic reservoir. However, it is imperative that the venous conduit retains its ability to distend while venoconstriction is mobilizing blood volume from the splanchnic capacitance. We believe this occurs by a combination of reduced adrenergic innervation in the conduit veins, increased adenosine activated vasodilator receptors in the conduit vein, and a dilatory IVC remodeling with aerobic endurance training [25–28]. This allows venous resistance to either reduce or remain unchanged during aerobic exercise [16].

Data on IVC remodeling can be inferred from studies of endurance trained athletes versus sedentary persons. One study established a 17% larger diameter taken from sequential long-axis view of the IVC in trained versus untrained females [28]. In a study investigating echocardiographic parameters in highly trained athletes, IVC diameter was markedly dilated ($p < 0.001$) as compared to healthy age and sex matched controls (2.34 ± 0.48 cm and 1.14 ± 0.13 cm, respectively). Right-ventricular dimensions and VO2 max of the athletes and controls had significant positive correlation to IVC size. Of note, swimmers were found to have the largest IVC diameters. It is undetermined whether this finding is attributed to increased venous return in the supine exercise positioning or elevated intrathoracic pressure due to breath holding techniques. Breath holding training may lead to elevated right ventricular pressures and subsequent IVC dilation. However, Goldhammer et al. also noted significantly higher IVC diameter in all athletes including swimmers, high jumpers, runners, volleyball, basketball, and soccer players [27]. We propose that these findings suggest there is a dilatory remodeling of the IVC in trained aerobic athletes.

In an additional study abstracting the role of Body Mass Index (BMI), venous resistance and cardiac filling, we found that increasing BMI was associated with decreasing IVC cross sectional area (CSA). In contrast, **Figure 1** shows the expected positive correlation between aortic CSA and BMI. Persons with normal BMI were able to increase their EVTI sequentially with intensifying exercise. Whereas, the elevated BMI group's EVTI remained unchanged throughout (**Figure 2**). An increase in vascular resistance was also observed within the elevated BMI group [29]. Both the decrease in EVTI and the increase in venous resistance in patients with elevated BMI point to a reduced ability to increase cardiac preload and EVTI with exercise in this group. We hypothesize that the increased BMI population, defined as >25, displays a more sedentary lifestyle with less physical fitness, contributing to negative remodeling of the IVC leading to maladaptive cardiac filling and function during exercise.

The utility of the increase of IVC diameters in athletes is of note. One of our recent studies demonstrates how IVC dilation leads to a decrease in venous resistance and increase in cardiac output. In fourteen healthy subjects, non-contrast CT was used to measure IVC cross-sectional area during passive leg elevation and supine cycling exercise. Scans were obtained at baseline, during leg elevation, and while subjects performed supine exercise at 50% and 90% of their maximal effort. IVC cross-sectional area increased with passive leg raises ($p < 0.001$) and with 50% maximal effort

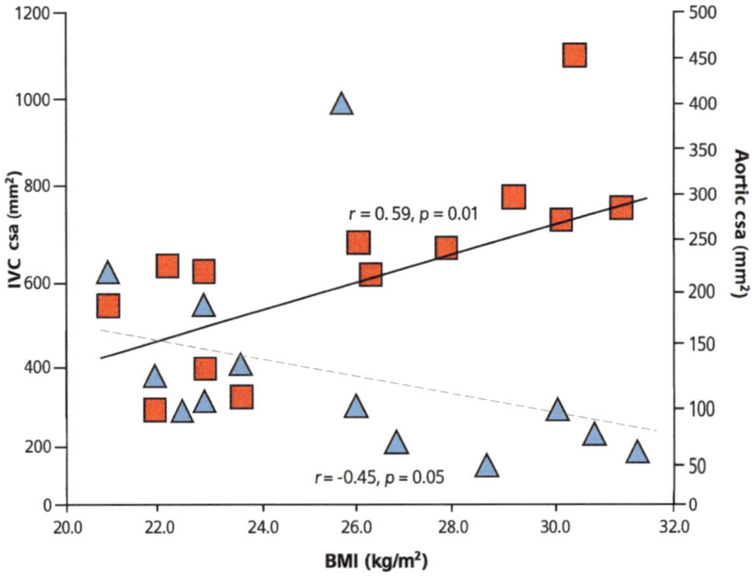

Figure 1.
Relationship of IVC CSA (blue) and aortic CSA (red) with body mass index (BMI). The figure depicts an inverse relationship between BMI and IVC CSA.

DOI: http://dx.doi.org/10.5772/intechopen.1012884

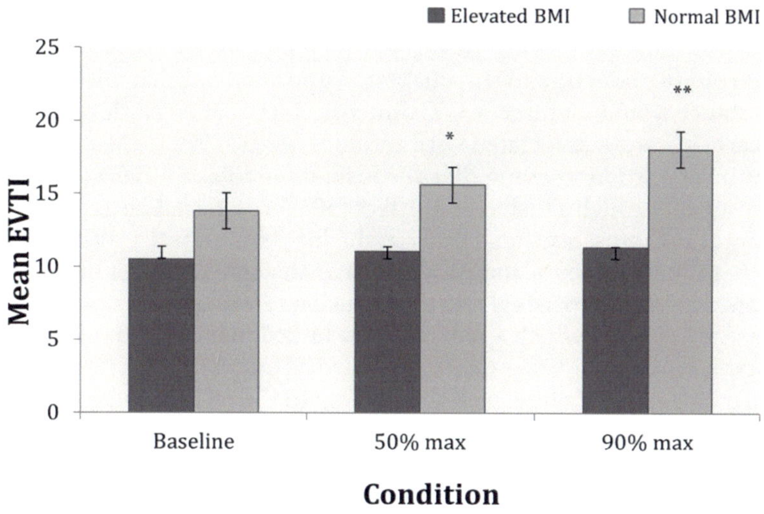

Figure 2.
*Mean E-wave Velocity Time Integral (EVTI) across intervention stages in normal and elevated BMI groups. A significant increase in early diastolic filling (EVTI) with incremental exercise is observed only in the normal BMI group (*p < 0.028; **p < 0.0019).*

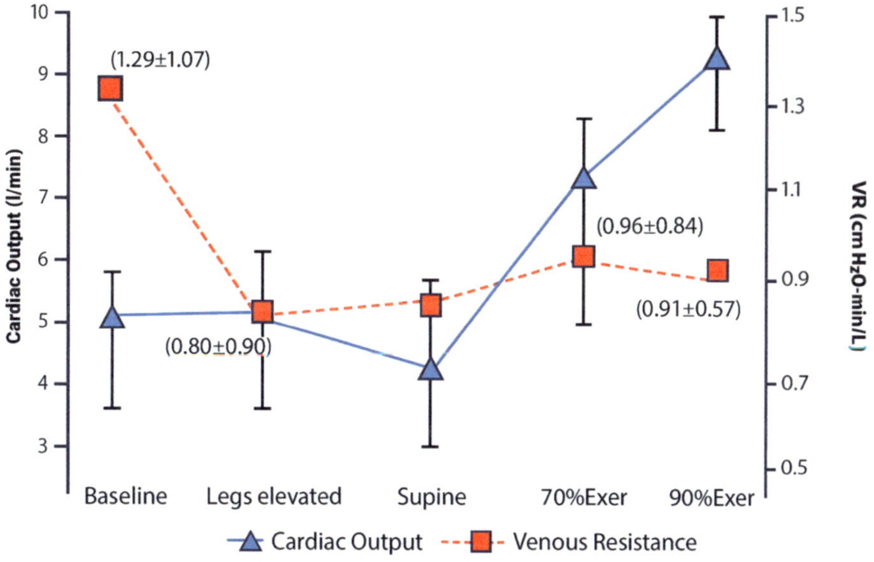

Figure 3.
Changes in cardiac output and venous resistance (VR) across different body positions and during exercise. Cardiac output presented with standard deviation error bars. VR displayed with numerical values. This figure shows that venous resistance reduces with passive leg elevation and remains reduced throughout increasing levels of supine exercise.

exercise ($p < 0.05$). **Figure 3** displays that as exercise effort intensified, cardiac output increased while venous resistance remained stable. This suggests increased IVC cross sectional area discouraged a rise in venous resistance during exercise [16].

Our observations support IVC remodeling as part of the training effect from repeated bouts of aerobic exercise. This facilitates increased venous return without any increasing resistance to venous blood flow.

2.4 Adenosine induced IVC dilation and increased cardiac output

Earlier in our introduction to this chapter, we pointed out that with laminar flow, venous resistance would increase if IVC dimensions remained static during the increased cardiac output associated with aerobic exercise. We are also aware of the Nussbacher investigation showing that adenosine was able to increase filling pressures in the heart solely through a lusiotropic effect [30]. We devised an experimental protocol looking at IVC cross sectional changes during a six-minute infusion of adenosine at 140 mcg/kg/min in patients undergoing pharmacologic stress for myocardial perfusion assessment. Surprisingly, at this infusion rate, adenosine provided a robust 63% increase in IVC CSA which appeared to be linked to increased mitral valve time velocity integral (MVTVI) times heart rate (cardiac output). Even more tightly correlated was the relative increase in cardiac output to the relative increase in IVC cross section within individuals (see **Figure 4**) [31]. Whether or not this occurs during human aerobic exercise is unknown. We do know that aerobic exercise increases the

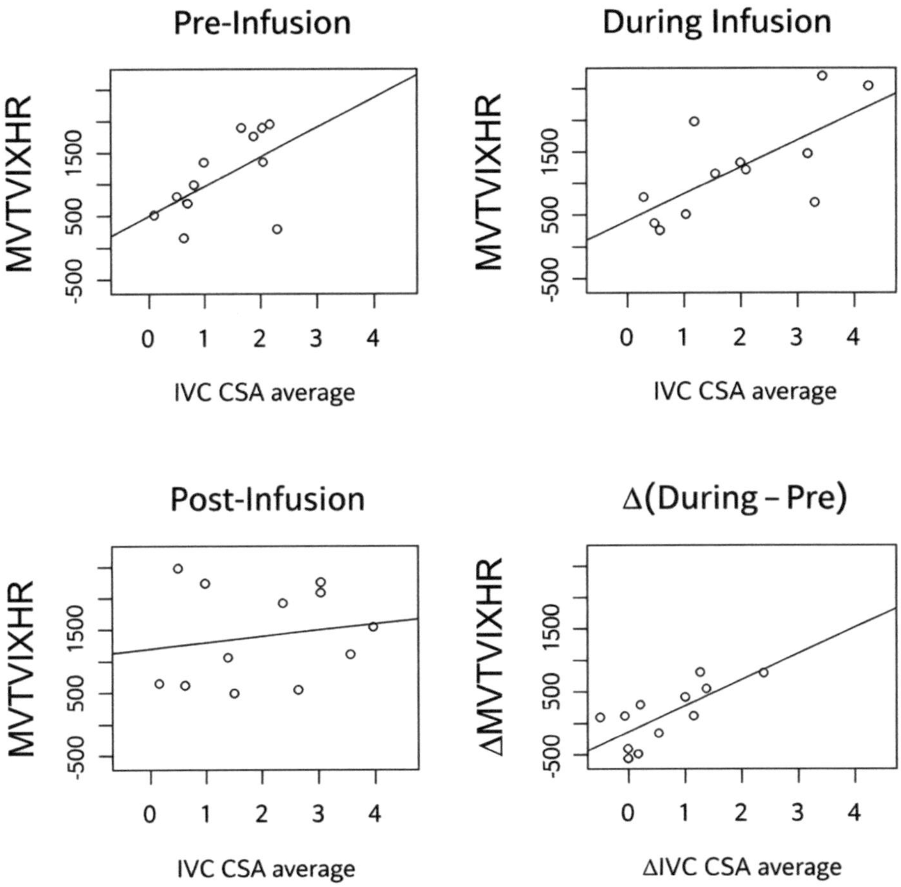

Figure 4.
Regression lines for MVTVI × HR versus IVC CSA average. Δ IVC CSA average = IVC CSA average during infusion – IVC CSA average pre-infusion. Δ MVTVI × HR = MVTVI × HR during infusion – MVTVI × HR pre-infusion. Note that change in IVC CSA is closely related to change in mitral valve time velocity integral (cardiac output) in final panel (r = 0.73, p = 0.006).

circulating adenosine levels effluxing from the heart by an almost three-fold increase over resting levels [32]. We are not aware of any human studies linking aerobic exercise to increased IVC adenosine levels associated with acute IVC dilation. Hence, although conceptually appealing, for adenosine induced IVC dilation as a means of reducing venous resistance during human aerobic exercise, no current experimental evidence exists. One should note however, that the problem of increasing IVC caliber during increased flow is elegantly managed via a remodeling of the IVC observed in elite aerobic athletes [27, 28]. This remodeling results in partially collapsed IVC at rest, which becomes more spherical (increased CSA) during aerobic exercise [29]. This remodeling results in passive increase in IVC CSA accommodating increased flow without any increase in venous resistance, as shown above in Section 2.3. Hence, we are aware that IVC caliber has the ability to increase in proportion to increased flows and prevent increase in venous resistance. There is good evidence pointing to IVC dilatory remodeling occurring in endurance athletes [27, 28]. Whether or not adenosine contributes to acute IVC dilation during aerobic exercise remains unproven at this time.

2.5 Cardiopulmonary circuit adaptations during aerobic exercise

Blood mobilization to the thoracic cavity during exercise increased cardiac output while increasing oxygen diffusion capacity. The low-pressure pulmonary circuit undergoes several adaptations under these conditions. Pulmonary transit time, referring to the time it takes blood to travel from the right to left sides of the heart, is a metric utilized to evaluate whole cardiopulmonary function. Several studies have demonstrated a significant decrease in pulmonary transit time during exercise. An instructive understanding of this relationship is derived from a study of patients with restrictive cardiomyopathy (RCM) which illustrated the relationship between pulmonary transit time and diastolic function. In this population, pulmonary transit time was significantly increased. More pertinent to our theories, pulmonary transit time increased with increasing stages of diastolic dysfunction, as seen in **Figure 5**.

Pulmonary transit times were correlated with echocardiographic doppler evaluation of diastolic function in these RCM patients. Thus, pulmonary transit time proves an effective qualitative measure of cardiopulmonary hemodynamics, specifically diastolic function and LV filling [33]. Measurement of pulmonary transit times using a first-pass radiotracer technique during rest and muscular exercise yielded that pulmonary transit times decreased by 55% when blood flow increased three-fold [34]. However, it appears that this adaptive mechanism reaches its limit at 2.5–3 times resting cardiac index [35]. These findings were confirmed in a study measuring pulmonary transit times and cardiac output in using a radiotracer technique and labeled blood boluses. The mean times decreased from 9.36 ± 1.41 seconds to less than 3 seconds during exercise [36]. Both studies suggest that the increased blood volume shunted to the thoracic circuit during aerobic exercise could result in improved function of the pulmonary vascular system by dilating the pulmonary conduit vessels leading to a decrease in pulmonary transit time.

As discussed previously, adenosine has proven its lusitropic properties in conduit vessels and coronary arteries. However, its dilatory effects have also been observed in the pulmonary arteries. In a study in patients with diagnosed pulmonary hypertension, adenosine infusions into the pulmonary artery yielded dose-dependent reduction in pulmonary artery pressure and increase in cardiac output. Mean pulmonary artery pressure decreased with statistical significance in all seven patients at the

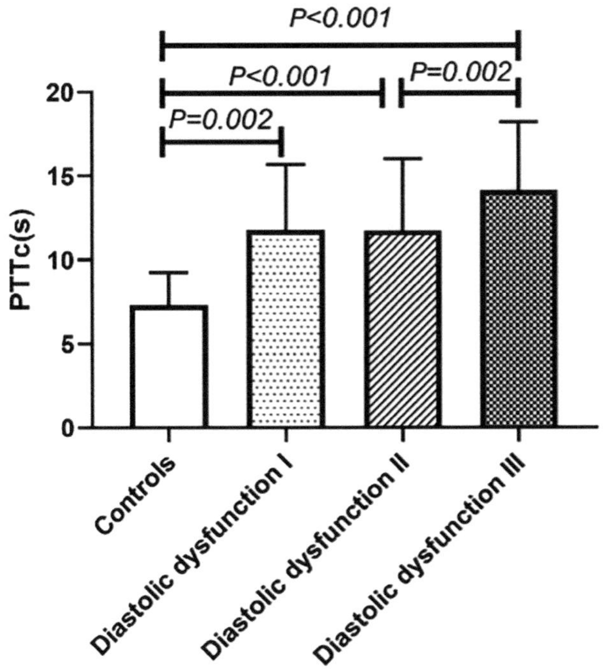

Figure 5.
Histograms depicting PTT vs. increasing grades of diastolic dysfunction (grade I–III). Note that as the degree of diastolic function increases, pulmonary transit time also increases.

highest dose of 0.05 mg/kg body wt/min for 10 minutes ($p < 0.001$). Cardiac output began its increase at the lowest dose, 0.01 mg/kg body wt/min for 10 minutes, with the maximum increase of 52.3% at 0.05 mg/kg/min ($p < 0.001$) [37].

Nussbacher et al. also discusses interesting effects of adenosine on the cardiopulmonary system. They describe an observed rise in pulmonary capillary wedge pressure (PCWP) with adenosine administration. PCWP often serves as an estimate of LAP and LVEDP to assess LV filling. The study investigated mechanisms for this increase in PCWP including alterations in left ventricular compliance, cardiac depression through a1 receptors, delayed cardiac relaxation, and altered vascular loading. Testing of these mechanisms was conducted through echocardiography of cardiac function. The study concluded that adenosine induction and rise in PCWP was not a result of worsening ventricular diastolic function. Chamber compliance, stiffness, isovolumic relaxation time, and thickness were not significantly changed by adenosine infusion. However, there was an observed increase in left and right heart filling, measured by LVEDP, LVEDV, and RAP. In conclusion, they suggest the possibility of an unexplored lusitropic effect of adenosine, altering vascular loading for improved LV filling and increased PCWP [30]. As detailed above, our study showed a 63% increase in IVC CSA with adenosine induction. This may serve as the explanation for the increase in PCWP observed by Nussbacher et al. It is clear that adenosine plays a role in vasodilating the pulmonary conduit vessels, mobilizing blood to the pulmonary vasculature, decreasing PTT, and improving diastolic flow into the left ventricle to improve cardiac output.

In conclusion, this section of our chapter has outlined the adaptations of the low-pressure system that occur during exercise, notably in major conduit veins and in the pulmonary arteries. These adaptations include dilation of the IVC, mobilization of blood volume from the splanchnic bed to the central compartment including pulmonary reservoir creation, and improved pulmonary transit. These studies also show the advantageous effects that these mechanisms have on diastolic filling and cardiac output, allowing successful aerobic exercise.

3. Cardiac adaptations facilitating diastolic function during aerobic exercise

In addition to adaptations within the low-pressure venous system, aerobic exercise triggers several important cardiac changes. One such response involves an increase in cardiac preload, initiated by an increase in venous return [26]. During aerobic exercise, the heart adapts to increased preload through both structural remodeling and functional changes. Notably, the key challenge during aerobic exercise is the reduction in diastolic duration, which results from prioritizing systolic ejection to ensure adequate systemic perfusion under higher metabolic demand [38]. As diastole shortens, the heart must respond with enhanced diastolic performance to maintain proper ventricular filling. Simultaneously, aerobic exercise promotes increased myocardial blood flow occurring during diastole and causes coronary vascular adaptations. These changes increase coronary perfusion during the shortened diastole, thereby supporting myocardial oxygen delivery and facilitating efficient diastolic function. This section highlights the myocardial, functional, and structural, as well as coronary vascular adaptations that collectively enhance diastolic function and lusitropy, enabling the heart to meet the increased oxygen demands resulting from aerobic exercise. The role of adenosine as a primary metabolic regulator of this process is discussed in more detail.

3.1 Mechanisms of functional myocardial adaptations during aerobic exercise

Cardiac muscle is unique in that, unlike the isotonic-isometric relaxation of skeletal muscle, it undergoes auxotonic relaxation. Auxotonic relaxation refers to the simultaneous change in load and length of cardiac muscle fibers [10]. This phenomenon enables the cardiac muscle to undergo force decline predominantly as the ventricular pressure falls, while the cardiac muscle fibers lengthen during rapid filling. Auxotonic relaxation is also load-dependent, meaning that as the load on the heart increases, it can adequately increase the degree to which it relaxes. This concept relates to a common method for assessing diastolic function: the E/A ratio. The variable E indicates the peak velocity of early, passive diastolic filling, and A represents the highest filling rate during atrial contraction [39]. Measured using echocardiography and Doppler during filling, the E/A ratio indicates how well the heart fills and relaxes during diastole. Similarly, the E/e′ ratio is used to assess diastolic function, where e′ is the early diastolic mitral annular tissue velocity. This technique helps understand LV filling pressures during diastole. Regarding cardiac adaptations during aerobic exercise, the E/A and E/e′ ratios change differently. The E/A ratio increases significantly as the heart improves early diastolic filling and becomes less dependent on blood volume from atrial contraction. The E/e′ ratio either remains unchanged or decreases as the heart maintains or lowers LV filling pressures. In other words, as ventricular filling increases with increasing early diastolic E wave filling, the mitral annulus motion must match this to maintain low diastolic pressures.

Expanding this discussion further than solely diastole, we can examine the effect of increased load on the myocardium in systole. Gaasch et al. detailed this concept in their work investigating the effect of additional loading of left ventricle while pressure is being generated on subsequent myocardial relaxation [40]. Utilizing an experimental method consisting of a computer-controlled servo pump connected to the left ventricle of a canine heart, they infused 6 mL of blood during early and late systole, while measuring the LV end systolic pressure as compared to controls. It was notable that the increase in load early in systole delayed the pressure decline, and in stark contrast the increased load late in systole led to a rapid decline in pressure. Delving deeper into the biochemical mechanism underlying this finding, these results can be explained through the actin-myosin crossbridge disengagement. Just prior to peak pressure generation, crossbridge engagement can be increased in response to a higher load. However, just after peak pressure generation, this is not the case and crossbridge disengagement occurs more rapidly, leading to a greater decrease in pressure. Therefore, these findings further exhibit the concept of "load-dependent relaxation" posited by Brutsaert [10] (**Figure 6**).

Fraites, Kass et al. focused their work on the E/A ratio as it relates to both diastolic function and chamber pressures [41]. The study was conducted using six isolated, blood-perfused canine hearts connected to an intracavitary volume servo-pump. A simulated atrial pressure waveform was employed to mimic diastolic filling, during which the E/A ratio was randomly set to 3:1, 1:1, or 1:3. Diastolic pressures were then measured at three distinct preload volumes. The key finding was that an E/A ratio of 3:1, representing predominant early diastolic filling, resulted in an early (first half) diastolic pressure increase that strongly correlated with the relaxation time constant ($r = 0.91, p < 0.0001$). This correlation was not observed with an E/A ratio of 1:3, representing predominant late diastolic filling ($p = 0.63$). Furthermore, at comparable

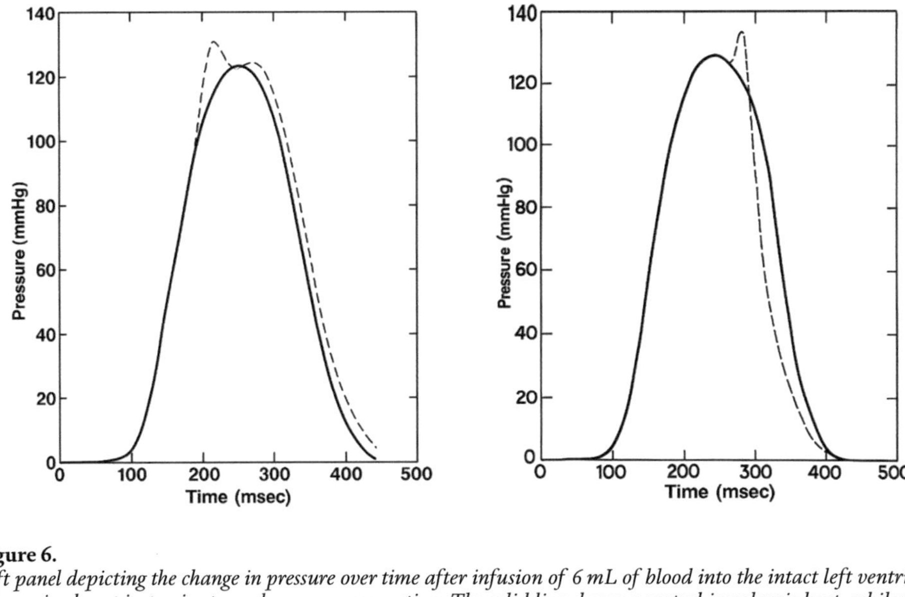

Figure 6.
Left panel depicting the change in pressure over time after infusion of 6 mL of blood into the intact left ventricle of a canine heart just prior to peak pressure generation. The solid line shows a control isovolumic beat, while the dashed line shows a beat following increased volume. The right panel demonstrates a change in pressure over time after infusion just after peak pressure generation. The peak negative dP/dt was much greater in the dashed line of the right panel (3.005 mmHg/s) as compared to the controls and the dashed line in the left panel (1.742 mmHg/s) Citation: Gaasch et. al [40].

ventricular volumes during the onset of viscous force decay, end-diastolic pressures were 37–50% lower with an E/A ratio of 3:1 compared to 1:3. These findings highlight the significant influence of myocardial viscoelasticity, defined as the heart's ability to resist deformation and restore its original geometry, on diastolic filling dynamics. Notably, these viscoelastic properties affect end-diastolic pressure independently of preload. As the E/A ratio declines due to impaired diastolic function, end-diastolic pressure rises accordingly. Therefore, diastolic performance may be optimized when a greater proportion of ventricular filling occurs during early diastole, consistent with pulmonary vasodilation, reduced pulmonary transit time, and improved E wave filling during aerobic exercise (**Figure 7**).

Burgess et al. focused their research on the E/e′ ratio, which helps improve understanding of diastolic function alongside E/A ratio values [44]. As explained earlier, the E/e′ ratio is valuable because it closely relates to the LV diastolic pressure. This is because the heart adjusts volume as it relaxes. The e′ variable is especially significant because it measures the rate of myocardial relaxation [44]. If the rate of early diastolic filling exceeds that of relaxation, it is reasonable to suggest that the pressure inside the LV will increase, and vice versa. This study aimed to measure the E/e′ ratio at rest and during exercise using an invasive technique. Thirty-seven patients participated in supine cycle ergometry, during which they underwent left heart catheterization. Separately, they measured the Doppler index of diastolic filling at rest and after exercise using a treadmill in 166 patients to explore the relationship between exercise capacity and E/e′ during exercise. They found a strong correlation between the E/e′ ratio and LVEDP at rest ($r = 0.67$) and during exercise ($r = 0.59$). Through receiver-operating curve analysis, they determined that a cutoff value of 13 for exercise E/e′ effectively identified patients with elevated LVEDP during exercise. These results show that individuals with higher LVEDP in response to aerobic exercise tend to have an increased E/e′ ratio, indicating impaired myocardial relaxation and worsened diastolic function.

Green et al. studied the cardiac functional adaptations to resistance and endurance training on 64 healthy individuals in a randomized crossover study [45]. One of their main goals was to understand the impact of both forms of exercise on diastolic function. To do so, they employed echocardiography and analyzed the E/e′ ratios of these participants. They saw that the E/e′ ratio improved and decreased following

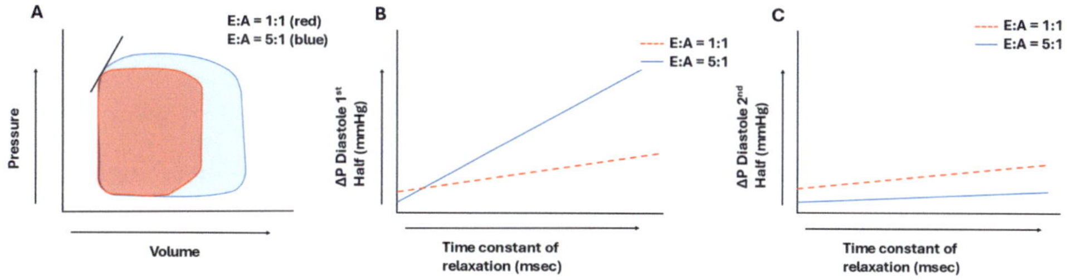

Figure 7.
Schematic interpretation of PV loops at rest and during exercise in endurance trained individuals and effects on diastolic pressures (authors developed hypothetical figure from observations derived by Fraites et al., Pelligrino et al., Aslanger et al.). A: Changes in pressure-volume loops in early and late diastole at rest (red) and during aerobic exercise (blue) in endurance trained individuals. Note the increased EDV and decreased EDP during exercise, resulting in increased stroke volume and stroke work. B: Rate of filling dependent pressure rise during the first half of diastole is greater during aerobic exercise due to the large volume of blood entering the ventricle during early diastole. C: No difference in rate of filling dependent pressure rise between rest and aerobic exercise in late diastole. However, there is significantly lower EDP when increased early diastolic filling has occurred. Hence, in endurance trained individuals, increasing blood volume during early diastole results in lower EDP [42, 43].

endurance training (**Δ**-0.35 ± 0.98, $p = 0.011$), while the ratio increased following resistance training (**Δ**0.35 ± 1.11, $p = 0.157$; $p = 0.001$ between modes of training). In the same vein as endurance training, Wasfy et al. investigated the cardiac adaptations to swim training in 17 collegiate swimmers after a 90-day period of intense training [46]. Their curiosity stemmed from the unique conditions swimming puts the body in as either the prone or supine position cause increased cardiac load volumes as compared to other endurance sports. Using transthoracic echocardiography, they found that, while the E/A ratio remained relatively unchanged, the peak average of both E ($p < 0.001$) and A increased ($p < 0.01$).

MacFarlane et al. researched the left ventricular structure and function among three groups of people: 10 elite endurance athletes (group 1), 10 elite weightlifters (group 2), and 10 inactive individuals (group 3) [47]. This study sought to elucidate the cardiac adaptations in a similar manner to the work done by Green et al., focusing on structural and functional changes. With regards to diastolic function, they measured the E/A ratio using Doppler echocardiography at rest and during exercise (cycling in the supine position). Their results demonstrated that the E/A ratio increased significantly in group 1 (3.37 ± 0.24) compared to groups 2 and 3 (2.38 ± 0.16 and 1.99 ± 0.10; $p < 0.003$). During exercise, the E/A ratio for group 1 was much higher than group 3 (1.95 ± 0.14 and 1.23 ± 0.05; $p < 0.001$), which also was the case when compared to group 2 (1.68 ± 0.15; p = ns). According to a recent study by Hoffmann et al., the E/A ratio recorded in endurance athletes and sprinters compared to resistance athletes such as throwers was significantly higher ($p < 0.01$). The E/e′ ratio was also affected and was significantly lower the endurance athletes in comparison to the resistance athletes ($p < 0.05$) [48].

Each of these studies detailed the benefits of aerobic exercise on the heart. Although they conducted their research under different conditions, they all share one common element: the improvement of diastolic function. The way we examine this improvement in diastole is influenced by the enhancement provided by auxotonic relaxation to improve early diastolic filling during a shortened diastolic phase. This phenomenon creates a physiological link between cardiac diastolic function during a period when diastolic filling time is significantly reduced. Hence, the increased venous return generated during aerobic exercise can fill the ventricle quicker and at lower filling pressures due to the mechanism of auxotonic relaxation.

3.2 Myocardial structural Remodeling to facilitate diastolic function during exercise

Sustained aerobic exercise drives a specific pattern of cardiac remodeling known as eccentric hypertrophy. This physiological adaptation features balanced increases in both left ventricular (LV) cavity size and wall thickness, enabling athletes to accommodate greater preload and augment stroke volume without compromising compliance or function [49]. These structural changes are mediated in part by the IGF-1/PI3K/Akt pathway, promoting cardiomyocyte growth in a non-fibrotic, symmetric manner that distinguishes it from pathological hypertrophy.

Echocardiographic studies provide evidence of sport- and training-specific remodeling. Among endurance athletes, particularly cyclists, increased LV end-diastolic diameters and wall thicknesses are well-documented, with cyclists demonstrating the most pronounced changes within this study relative to soccer players and long distance runners [50]. Basketball players, who engage in both aerobic and anaerobic activities, also exhibit moderate increases in LV mass and wall thickness.

These changes scale appropriately with body surface area and training intensity, suggesting physiological adaptation rather than a disease process [51].

Prospective training studies have confirmed that these structural changes can emerge within weeks to months of endurance conditioning. In a 90-day longitudinal study, endurance training led to significant increases in LV mass and volume, reinforcing the causal role of chronic volume overload in driving eccentric remodeling [52]. Right ventricular changes parallel those of the left heart. Endurance athletes show increased RV diastolic dimensions and enhanced systolic and diastolic performance, while strength-trained athletes exhibit minimal RV change [50, 52].

In addition to ventricular remodeling, atrial adaptations are also common. Left atrial (LA) enlargement occurs in response to increased preload and is often seen in both endurance athletes and basketball players [50, 51]. This enlargement supports efficient diastolic filling and is considered benign in the athletic context. This physiological adaptation contrasts with pathological LA remodeling associated with an increased risk of atrial fibrillation. Right atrial (RA) dilation, though less studied, is also recognized in endurance athletes with concurrent right ventricular (RV) remodeling [53]. Together, these adaptations represent a global cardiac response to chronic hemodynamic stress.

Functionally, these morphological changes preserve or enhance diastolic performance. Endurance athletes and cyclists typically demonstrate elevated E/A ratios, reflecting robust early filling, alongside preserved or low E/e′ ratios indicating normal LV filling pressures [48, 50, 54]. These parameters help distinguish physiologic remodeling from diastolic dysfunction.

Sport-specific differences further support the training-induced nature of remodeling. Cyclists exhibit the most pronounced left and right ventricular and atrial dilation, followed by soccer players, runners, and basketball players. Throwers show minimal remodeling, reinforcing the principle that sustained volume load, not intermittent pressure load, drives structural changes [48, 50, 51].

Distinguishing physiological from pathological hypertrophy is an important distinction in clinical settings. Athlete's heart is characterized by symmetric enlargement, preserved systolic and diastolic function, absence of fibrosis, and reversibility with deconditioning [54–56]. For example, athlete's heart may mimic hypertrophic cardiomyopathy (HCM) on echocardiography, but regression of LV thickness with detraining supports a physiological origin, whereas HCM shows persistent hypertrophy with associated fibrosis.

In summary, endurance training appears to enhance ventricular size without interfering with rapid relaxation properties of an intact auxotonic relaxation mechanism. If the athlete performs extensive isometric loading, it can lead to associated concentric hypertrophy, which can then create problems determining if it is pathologic or physiologic in origin. The benefit of overall ventricular dilation is obvious in its ability to increase end diastolic volume, which will lead to an increase in stroke volume, and reduce dependence on increased heart rate, to support increase in cardiac output.

3.3 Coronary vascular mechanism to facilitate diastolic function during exercise

While functional and structural remodeling of the heart occurs in response to aerobic exercise, manifesting as improved chamber compliance, better diastolic filling, and myocardial hypertrophy, these changes are accompanied by increased energy demands. Myocardial relaxation, in particular, is an active process that requires significant energy [57]. On the molecular level, relaxation mainly involves the active reuptake of cytosolic calcium into the sarcoplasmic reticulum through the sarco/endoplasmic reticulum Ca^{2+}-ATPase (SERCA), a process closely linked to ATP availability. Because ATP is mostly produced through oxidative phosphorylation, the heart's ability to relax efficiently depends on sufficient oxygen delivery. This dependence on oxidative metabolism underscores the essential role of coronary circulation in supporting exercise-induced cardiac adaptations. As the heart undergoes structural and functional changes, a parallel set of vascular adaptations must occur to meet the increased oxygen demands. Specifically, improvements in coronary blood flow, both at rest and during exertion, become critical to ensure sufficient myocardial oxygenation. Thus, the enhancement of coronary vascular function represents a fundamental component of the integrated cardiovascular response to aerobic exercise, directly supporting the metabolic and mechanical requirements of the remodeled myocardium.

White et al. focused their investigation on how exercise training affects the capillaries and arterioles of the heart [58]. They specifically studied these effects in minipigs, which underwent exercise training by running on a treadmill and had data recorded at 1, 3, 8, and 16 weeks compared to controls. Measuring the capillary and arteriolar densities of the epicardial vessels, their team observed that the maximum O_2 consumption increased steadily as the study progressed. They divided the arterioles into five groups based on diameter. At the end of the study, the number of arterioles and the diameter of larger vessels had increased. These changes led to a 37% increase in the total vascular bed cross-sectional area. Ultimately, they suggest that the new capillaries formed and then developed into small arterioles, indicating that capillary angiogenesis in response to aerobic exercise could serve as a source of increased coronary blood flow.

Hotta et al. sought to elucidate whether coronary microvascular dysfunction plays a role in age-related diastolic dysfunction and if aerobic exercise can reverse these changes in rats [59]. They compared young and old rats before and after they took part in exercise training to sedentary controls. The main variables that were measured included isovolumic relaxation time, early diastolic filling (E/A ratio), myocardial performance index, aortic stiffness (pulse wave velocity), and most importantly for our purposes: coronary blood flow and coronary arteriolar vasodilation. They observed a decrease in coronary blood flow and endothelium dependent vasodilation in older sedentary rats as compared to younger ones both at rest and during exercise. In addition, exercise training was seen to completely reverse the impairments in coronary blood flow and endothelium-dependent vasodilation. These findings, combined with the reversal of a decrease in E/A ratio, support the role of aerobic exercise augmenting coronary vasculature function to improve diastolic function in older rats.

Collectively, aerobic exercise causes coordinated adaptations in the heart muscle and coronary vessels that support improved diastolic function. Enhanced coronary blood flow ensures sufficient oxygen delivery to meet the increased metabolic needs of the remodeled heart. While these structural and functional changes are well-documented, our understanding of the molecular mechanisms underlying these adaptations remains limited. The following section will explore the key molecular regulators that coordinate the integrated coronary vascular response to exercise.

3.4 Role of adenosine in modulating coronary circulation

As aerobic exercise increases myocardial workload, the energy needs of diastole rise significantly, especially in an athlete's hypertrophied heart. In these conditions, metabolic feedback mechanisms play a crucial role in enhancing coronary blood flow to meet the increased demand. Among these, adenosine, a purine nucleoside produced from ATP breakdown during periods of high metabolic stress, acts as a key mediator. During exercise, faster ATP turnover causes intracellular AMP buildup and subsequent extracellular adenosine formation through ecto-5′-nucleotidase, closely matching myocardial energy demand [60]. These observations highlight adenosine's pivotal role as a metabolic regulator that links increased myocardial energy demand with adaptive coronary vasodilation, making it a key contributor to exercise-induced improvements in cardiac perfusion and diastolic function.

Adenosine, as one of the key regulators of myocardial perfusion, has been of interest for decades due to its ability to influence coronary artery vasomotor function. The main aspect that has been extensively studied is its potent vasodilatory effect on the coronary vessels. As early as the 1920s, studies showed that injecting adenosine into the superior vena cava causes an increase in coronary blood flow, as measured in the coronary sinus of dogs' hearts [14]. Specifically, a dose of 10 mg of adenosine increased flow from 41 cc per minute to 200 cc per minute. This was especially notable because the dilation was comparable to the then-standard vasodilator, sodium nitrite. Studies have also documented a decrease in arterial pressure in response to adenosine. Further investigation revealed that the pressure drop (~50 mmHg) could not be entirely attributed to reduced heart rate, as a 40 mg infusion of adenosine into the aorta of a 6 kg dog, without affecting cardiac conduction time, still lowered arterial pressure (~25 mmHg) [14]. Therefore, it was concluded that coronary vasodilation caused by adenosine must also contribute to the decrease in arterial pressure. This is evident when observing an increase in pulmonary pressure during adenosine administration, which dilates the coronary vessels that link the systemic and pulmonary circulations.

In the 1960s, Robert Berne sought to elucidate the mechanism through which the myocardium responds to hypoxia [13]. He hypothesized that the degradation of adenosine into inosine and hypoxanthine potentially indicated an increased metabolic demand of the myocardium under this condition. In a series of carefully designed experiments, Berne sought to elucidate the role of adenosine as a key metabolic regulator of coronary blood flow. His investigations began with isolated cat hearts perfused using a Langendorff preparation under hypoxic conditions. He observed a marked increase in coronary blood flow accompanied by elevated levels of inosine and hypoxanthine, adenine nucleotide metabolites formed during ATP degradation. Importantly, these levels returned to baseline upon reoxygenation, suggesting that hypoxia stimulates endogenous adenosine production, which acts as a coronary vasodilator to restore oxygen balance. To extend these findings in a more physiologic setting, Berne studied anesthetized dogs undergoing thoracotomy, with cannulation of the left coronary artery and coronary sinus. Induction of partial asphyxia through reduced respiratory volume led to similar increases in inosine and hypoxanthine concentrations in the coronary sinus, along with enhanced coronary blood flow. In contrast, these metabolites were nearly absent in arterial blood, reinforcing their local myocardial origin in response to metabolic stress. Further, constriction of coronary vessels triggered a reactive increase in flow, consistent with the presence of locally acting vasodilators. Berne then directly tested the vasodilatory effect of adenosine itself by infusing it into the left coronary artery. This intervention led to a doubling of coronary blood flow, an effect that was reversed by restricting the inflow. Notably, in this setting, inosine and hypoxanthine were not detected in the coronary sinus, likely because exogenous adenosine bypasses ATP breakdown and acts directly on coronary vasculature. Taken together, these early studies provided compelling evidence that adenosine, generated during states of increased myocardial energy demand, serves as a critical endogenous modulator that couples metabolic stress to coronary vasodilation.

Substantial experimental evidence has now established adenosine as a key regulator of cardiovascular function and coronary vasomotor tone. Its role in coupling myocardial metabolic demand to local blood flow is well characterized, and the molecular mechanisms underlying its action have been increasingly clarified [61–66]. Adenosine is released from the cardiac myocytes through nucleoside transporters and activates membrane adenosine receptors (A_1, A_{2B} and A_{2A}) on vascular smooth muscle and endothelium to exert potent vasodilatory effects, facilitating relaxation of the coronary microvasculature [63, 64, 66]. In endothelial cells, adenosine has been shown to activate endothelial nitric oxide synthase, leading to nitric oxide production [61, 62]. This effect is significant during the post-exercise recovery period, when elevated adenosine concentrations persist and continue to regulate perfusion [60]. In addition to its hemodynamic actions, adenosine promotes angiogenesis, contributing to long-term microvascular remodeling. Experimental models employing dipyridamole, an adenosine reuptake inhibitor, have demonstrated that chronically elevated adenosine levels stimulate vascular proliferation even under normoxic conditions [60].

These experimental insights not only establish adenosine as a critical mediator of coronary vasoregulation but also set the stage for understanding its broader role in driving exercise-induced cardiovascular adaptations, including enhanced myocardial perfusion, improved endothelial function, and augmented coronary vascularization.

3.5 Competing mediators of coronary metabolic adaptation of aerobic exercise

Although adenosine's coronary vasodilatory properties are widely accepted, its role as a principal regulator of coronary blood flow during exercise subject to competing interpretations. Tune et al. demonstrated that coronary hyperemia during treadmill exercise in dogs was preserved despite adenosine receptor blockade, suggesting adenosine is not required for local metabolic control under physiological conditions [65]. Their findings implied that alternative pathways may be sufficient to meet myocardial oxygen demands during exercise. In contrast, Duncker et al.'s experiments, also using dog models, support a conditional role for adenosine [67, 68]. They demonstrated that while adenosine may not be dominant under normal circumstances, it becomes functionally critical when other vasodilatory pathways, such as K-ATP channels, are inhibited. Specifically, when K-ATP channels were pharmacologically blocked, adenosine receptor antagonism significantly attenuated exercise-induced coronary vasodilation, indicating that adenosine acts as a compensatory vasodilator under conditions of restricted metabolic flexibility or flow reserve.

Other experiments by Barron et al., using porcine carotid artery preparations, revealed that exposure to adenosine increased oxygen consumption by approximately 52%, accompanied by significant increases in intracellular ATP, phosphocreatine, and total adenine nucleotide content. These changes indicated an active upregulation of mitochondrial metabolism rather than passive changes in tone. Furthermore, partial inhibition of the vasodilatory response by glibenclamide suggests involvement of ATP-sensitive potassium channels. Notably, these effects were reduced under hypoxic conditions, emphasizing that adenosine's metabolic feedback loop depends on adequate oxygen availability [69].

Chronic endurance training appears to amplify adenosine-mediated pathways. In a 10-week swimming protocol involving normotensive rats, significant increases in coronary blood flow and myocardial capillary-to-fiber ratio were observed. These adaptations were accompanied by the upregulation of CD39 (E-NTPDase1) and CD73 (ecto-5′-nucleotidase), key enzymes in the extracellular ATP-to-adenosine cascade. Enhanced adenosine hydrolysis was observed in both circulating serum and myocardial tissue, suggesting a coordinated systemic and local enhancement in adenosinergic signaling capacity [70].

Additional mediators such as hydrogen peroxide (H_2O_2) and nitric oxide (NO) have been implicated in coronary vasodilation during increased cardiac metabolic demand. Yada et al. demonstrated that H_2O_2 plays a crucial role in pacing-induced metabolic vasodilation, reinforcing the idea that multiple redundant and interacting pathways regulate coronary blood flow [71]. These findings suggest that the coronary microvasculature relies on a network of signaling molecules, with adenosine serving as one of several dynamically recruited mediators, depending on the prevailing physiologic or pathophysiologic context.

Taken together, these findings highlight the important role of adenosine in regulating coronary blood flow during exercise. Adenosine appears to serve as a key compensatory vasodilator, especially when other mechanisms are compromised or when metabolic demands are exceptionally high. Its interplay with pathways such as K-ATP channels, mitochondrial metabolism, and nitric oxide signaling underscores its integration into a broader, redundant regulatory network that ensures adequate myocardial perfusion. Moreover, chronic endurance training enhances the adenosinergic system through upregulation of enzymatic components involved in ATP breakdown, suggesting an adaptive augmentation of this pathway with repeated exercise. These insights position adenosine not as a sole regulator, but as a flexible and critical contributor to the finely tuned orchestration of coronary vascular adaptations to exercise (**Figure 8**).

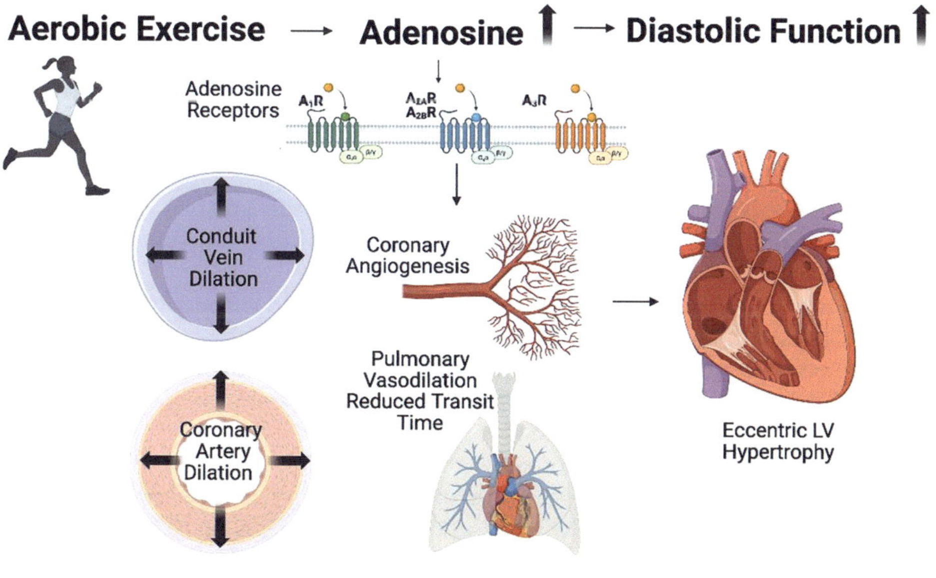

Figure 8.
Schema of proposed mechanisms by which adenosine facilitates LV diastolic function to adapt to aerobic exercise. Created by authors with BioRender.com.

4. Aerobic endurance training to improve diastolic function in chronic disease states

The benefits of aerobic endurance training seem to be transferable to improving diastolic function in other chronic disease states. Edelmann et al. showed that with a group of patients with diastolic heart failure, that 3 months of supervised endurance/resistance training, resulted in an improvement in diastolic function measured by a decreased E/e′ ratio ($p < 0.001$) and left atrial volume index ($p < 0.001$) [72]. Chaveles et al., in a smaller study, found a more modest improvement ($p < 0.05$). It appears that the improvement in diastolic function induced by aerobic endurance training is applicable to other disease states but requires continued endurance training to maintain the benefits [73].

5. Limitations

In this chapter we have highlighted the potential mechanisms for improving diastolic function during aerobic exercise, based on available conceptual studies. Unfortunately, we do not have many clinical studies to support the putative diastolic enhancements which occur with aerobic exercise and training. We have tried to point out where data is sparse or missing. We hope that this chapter will serve to stimulate the performance of more robust studies to confirm or refute the implied mechanisms for enhancing diastolic function through aerobic exercise presented in this chapter.

6. Conclusion

By virtue of the exponential reduction in diastolic filling time during aerobic exercise, achievement of aerobic athletic performance is a challenge that can only be surmounted with drastically improved diastolic filling. We present a comprehensive construct from venous capacitance mobilization to conduit vein dilation, to pulmonary transit enhancement, ending with activation of cardiac auxotonic relaxation and expansion of coronary vascular substrate delivery capabilities. We believe that this chapter should encourage further research into the mechanisms, extent, and limitations of diastolic enhancement during aerobic exercise. In fact, it has become common knowledge that the difference between elite aerobic athletes and sedentary individuals is the ability to achieve major enhancement of diastolic function during aerobic exercise.

We present a comprehensive role for adenosine mediated vasodilation in enhancing diastolic function in the low-pressure compartment and pulmonary vasculature. This complements the well-known cardiac effects of adenosine as the metabolic regulator of coronary blood flow and perfusion. These observations serve to strengthen the perception that adenosine is the endogenous enhancer of diastolic function and aerobic exercise in humans. Auxotonic relaxation allows rapid diastolic filling, and its impairment is the first sign of diastolic dysfunction. Eccentric hypertrophy develops with aerobic training, preserves the auxotonic relaxation mechanism, and further enhances the ability to increase cardiac output with aerobic exercise in athletes. The ideas presented in this chapter have not all been rigorously, scientifically confirmed, but we hope that our chapter will prompt a reexamination of the mechanisms that underlie the optimization of diastolic function during aerobic exercise in humans.

Acknowledgements

The authors would like to acknowledge John V Tyberg, MD, PhD (deceased) and Otto Smiseth, MD, PhD, who introduced the authors to the scientific questions and acute adaptations inherent to the low-pressure cardiovascular system. We would also like to acknowledge the Alberta Heritage Foundation for Medical Research (AHFMR) and the University of Calgary/Foothills Hospital for providing the means to allow VJBR to initiate experimental studies of the low-pressure compartment. Special thanks to Mark Schwade, MD, for his technical support.

Conflict of interest

The authors declare no conflict of interest.

Author details

Vincent J.B. Robinson[1*], Soham Kulkarni[2], Rohan Sharma[1], Thomas Hornaday[1], Ensley Tanner[2], Kuang-Drew Li[2], Tathya Patel[2], Rajavi Solanki[3], Hannah Griffin[2*] and Zsolt Bagi[4]

1 Division of Cardiology, Department of Medicine, Medical College of Georgia at Augusta University, Augusta, GA, USA

2 Medical College of Georgia at Augusta University, Augusta, GA, USA

3 Independent Researcher

4 Department of Physiology, Medical College of Georgia at Augusta University, Augusta, GA, USA

*Address all correspondence to: vrobinso@augusta.edu and hgriffin3@augusta.edu

References

[1] Warburton DE, Nicol CW, Bredin SS. Health benefits of physical activity: The evidence. CMAJ. 2006;**174**(6):801-809

[2] Patel H, Alkhawam H, Madanieh R, Shah N, Kosmas CE, Vittorio TJ. Aerobic vs anaerobic exercise training effects on the cardiovascular system. World Journal of Cardiology. 2017;**9**(2):134-138

[3] Kim MH, Sung JH, Jin MN, Jang E, Yu HT, Kim TH, et al. Impact of physical activity on all-cause mortality according to specific cardiovascular disease. Frontiers in Cardiovascular Medicine. 2022;**9**:811058

[4] Elgaddal N, Kramarow EA, Reuben C. Physical activity among adults aged 18 and over: United States, 2020. NCHS Data Brief. 2022;**443**:1-8

[5] Whelton SP, Chin A, Xin X, He J. Effect of aerobic exercise on blood pressure: A meta-analysis of randomized, controlled trials. Annals of Internal Medicine. 2002;**136**(7):493-503

[6] Sequeira V, van der Velden J. Historical perspective on heart function: The Frank-Starling Law. Biophysical Reviews. 2015;**7**(4):421-447

[7] Joyner MJ, Casey DP. Regulation of increased blood flow (hyperemia) to muscles during exercise: A hierarchy of competing physiological needs. Physiological Reviews. 2015;**95**(2):549-601

[8] Guyton AC, Lindsey AW, Abernathy B, Langston JB. Mechanism of the increased venous return and cardiac output caused by epinephrine. The American Journal of Physiology. 1958;**192**(1):126-130

[9] King J, Lowery DR. Physiology, Cardiac Output. Treasure Island (FL): StatPearls; 2025

[10] Brutsaert DL, Sys SU. Relaxation and diastole of the heart. Physiological Reviews. 1989;**69**(4):1228-1315

[11] Fagard R. Athlete's heart. Heart. 2003;**89**(12):1455-1461

[12] Mills JD, Moore GE, Thompson PD. The athlete's heart. Clinics in Sports Medicine. 1997;**16**(4):725-737

[13] Berne RM. Cardiac nucleotides in hypoxia: Possible role in regulation of coronary blood flow. The American Journal of Physiology. 1963;**204**:317-322

[14] Drury AN, Szent-Gyorgyi A. The physiological activity of adenine compounds with especial reference to their action upon the mammalian heart. The Journal of Physiology. 1929;**68**(3):213-237

[15] Greenway CV, Lautt WW. Blood volume, the venous system, preload, and cardiac output. Canadian Journal of Physiology and Pharmacology. 1986;**64**(4):383-387

[16] Robinson V, Krothapalli S, Saleem U, Mandawat M, Corley J, Halbert J, et al. The hemodynamics of inferior vena cava caliber changes from rest to exercise. Archives of General Internal Medicine. 2018;**2**(1):20-25

[17] Greenway CV, Lister GE. Capacitance effects and blood reservoir function in the splanchnic vascular bed during non-hypotensive haemorrhage and blood volume expansion in anaesthetized cats. The Journal of Physiology. 1974;**237**(2):279-294

[18] Hayashi N, Yamaoka-Endo M, Someya N, Fukuba Y. Blood flow in non-muscle tissues and organs during exercise: Nature of splanchnic and ocular circulation. The Journal of Physical Fitness and Sports Medicine. 2012;**1**(2):281-286

[19] Fudim M, Kaye David M, Borlaug Barry A, Shah Sanjiv J, Rich S, Kapur Navin K, et al. Venous tone and stressed blood volume in heart failure. JACC. 2022;**79**(18):1858-1869

[20] Patel RB, Shah SJ. The splanchnic reservoir: An oasis for blood volume in heart failure with preserved ejection fraction? European Journal of Heart Failure. 2021;**23**(7):1144-1146

[21] Flamm SD, Taki J, Moore R, Lewis SF, Keech F, Maltais F, et al. Redistribution of regional and organ blood volume and effect on cardiac function in relation to upright exercise intensity in healthy human subjects. Circulation. 1990;**81**(5):1550-1559

[22] Musch TI, Friedman DB, Pitetti KH, Haidet GC, Stray-Gundersen J, Mitchell JH, et al. Regional distribution of blood flow of dogs during graded dynamic exercise. Journal of Applied Physiology (1985). 1987;**63**(6):2269-2277

[23] McAllister RM. Adaptations in control of blood flow with training: Splanchnic and renal blood flows. Medicine and Science in Sports and Exercise. 1998;**30**(3):375-381

[24] Braunwald E, Kelly ER. The effects of exercise on central blood volume in man. The Journal of Clinical Investigation. 1960;**39**(2):413-419

[25] Nilsson H. Adrenergic nervous control of resistance and capacitance vessels. Studies on isolated blood vessels from the rat. Acta Physiologica Scandinavica. Supplementum. 1985;**541**:1-34

[26] Robinson VJBCL, Mehta V, Oribabor C. Dynamic Adaptations in the Human Low-Pressure Compartment Facilitating Cardiovascular Responses at Rest and Exercise. Hemodynamics of the Human Body. London, UK: IntechOpen; 2024

[27] Goldhammer E, Mesnick N, Abinader EG, Sagiv M. Dilated inferior vena cava: A common echocardiographic finding in highly trained elite athletes. Journal of the American Society of Echocardiography. 1999;**12**(11):988-993

[28] Hedman K, Nylander E, Henriksson J, Bjarnegard N, Brudin L, Tamas E. Echocardiographic characterization of the inferior vena cava in trained and untrained females. Ultrasound in Medicine & Biology. 2016;**42**(12):2794-2802

[29] Kapuku GK, Krothapalli SM, Corley JH, Saleem U, Mandawat MK, Halbert JD, et al. Role of BMI and venous resistance in modulation of cardiac filling. Archives of General Internal Medicine. 2018;**2**(1):26-31

[30] Nussbacher A, Arie S, Kalil R, Horta P, Feldman MD, Bellotti G, et al. Mechanism of adenosine-induced elevation of pulmonary capillary wedge pressure in humans. Circulation. 1995;**92**(3):371-379

[31] Majidi FVMC, Hreibe H, Mahbub F, Corley JH, Mandawat M, et al. Adenosine induces dilation of the inferior vena cava and increases transmitral flow. Journal of the American College of Cardiology. 2010;**55**(10A):1-19

[32] Watkinson WP, Foley DH, Rubio R, Berne RM. Myocardial adenosine formation with increased

cardiac performance in the dog. The American Journal of Physiology. 1979;**236**(1):H13-H21

[33] Gao Y, Min CY, Jiang YN, Shi R, Guo YK, Xu HY, et al. Association of pulmonary transit time and pulmonary blood volume from first-pass perfusion cardiac MRI with diastolic dysfunction and left ventricle deformation in restrictive cardiomyopathy. Journal of Magnetic Resonance Imaging. 2024;**60**(6):2343-2355

[34] Kuikka JT. Effect of increasing blood flow on distribution of pulmonary transit times in man. Physiological Measurement. 2000;**21**(2):241-250

[35] Zavorsky GS, Walley KR, Russell JA. Red cell pulmonary transit times through the healthy human lung. Experimental Physiology. 2003;**88**(2):191-200

[36] Hopkins SR, Belzberg AS, Wiggs BR, McKenzie DC. Pulmonary transit time and diffusion limitation during heavy exercise in athletes. Respiration Physiology. 1996;**103**(1):67-73

[37] Morgan JM, McCormack DG, Griffiths MJ, Morgan CJ, Barnes PJ, Evans TW. Adenosine as a vasodilator in primary pulmonary hypertension. Circulation. 1991;**84**(3):1145-1149

[38] Gledhill N, Cox D, Jamnik R. Endurance athletes' stroke volume does not plateau: Major advantage is diastolic function. Medicine and Science in Sports and Exercise. 1994;**26**(9):1116-1121

[39] Kass DA. Assessing and interpreting diastolic function in animal models of heart disease. Journal of Molecular and Cellular Cardiology. 2024;**197**:1-4

[40] Gaasch WH, Blaustein AS, Bing OH. Asynchronous (segmental early) relaxation of the left ventricle. Journal of the American College of Cardiology. 1985;**5**(4):891-897

[41] Fraites TJ Jr, Saeki A, Kass DA. Effect of altering filling pattern on diastolic pressure-volume curve. Circulation. 1997;**96**(12):4408-4414

[42] Aslanger E, Assous B, Bihry N, Beauvais F, Logeart D, Cohen-Solal A. Effects of cardiopulmonary exercise rehabilitation on left ventricular mechanical efficiency and ventricular-arterial coupling in patients with systolic heart failure. Journal of the American Heart Association. 2015;**4**(10):e002084

[43] Pellegrino A, Toncelli L, Vanni S, Modesti A, Pedrizzetti G, Modesti PA. Structural and functional remodeling for elite cyclists during exercise; pressure-volume loops and hemodynamic forces analysis. American Journal of Physiology. Heart and Circulatory Physiology. 2025;**328**(3):H393-H400

[44] Burgess MI, Jenkins C, Sharman JE, Marwick TH. Diastolic stress echocardiography: Hemodynamic validation and clinical significance of estimation of ventricular filling pressure with exercise. Journal of the American College of Cardiology. 2006;**47**(9):1891-1900

[45] Green DJ, Marsh CE, Thomas HJ, Maslen BA, Collis J, Lester L, et al. Cardiac functional adaptation to resistance and endurance exercise training: A randomized crossover study. American Journal of Physiology. Heart and Circulatory Physiology. 2024;**326**(4):H929-HH37

[46] Wasfy MM, Weiner RB, Wang F, Berkstresser B, Deluca J, Hutter AM Jr, et al. Myocardial adaptations to competitive swim training. Medicine and Science in Sports and Exercise. 2019;**51**(10):1987-1994

[47] MacFarlane N, Northridge DB, Wright AR, Grant S, Dargie HJ. A comparative study of left ventricular structure and function in elite athletes. British Journal of Sports Medicine. 1991;**25**(1):45-48

[48] Hoffmann F, Moestl S, Wooten SV, Stray-Gundersen S, Tomczak CR, Tank J, et al. Left ventricular dimensions and diastolic function are different in throwers, endurance athletes, and sprinters from the world masters athletics championships. Frontiers in Physiology. 2021;**12**:643764

[49] Furrer R, Hawley JA, Handschin C. The molecular athlete: Exercise physiology from mechanisms to medals. Physiological Reviews. 2023;**103**(3):1693-1787

[50] Moro AS, Okoshi MP, Padovani CR, Okoshi K. Doppler echocardiography in athletes from different sports. Medical Science Monitor. 2013;**19**:187-193

[51] Engel DJ, Schwartz A, Homma S. Athletic cardiac Remodeling in US professional basketball players. JAMA Cardiology. 2016;**1**(1):80-87

[52] Baggish AL, Wang F, Weiner RB, Elinoff JM, Tournoux F, Boland A, et al. Training-specific changes in cardiac structure and function: A prospective and longitudinal assessment of competitive athletes. Journal of Applied Physiology. 2008;**104**(4):1121-1128

[53] D'Ascenzi F, Anselmi F, Focardi M, Mondillo S. Atrial enlargement in the Athlete's heart: Assessment of atrial function may help distinguish adaptive from pathologic remodeling. Journal of the American Society of Echocardiography. 2018;**31**(2):148-157

[54] Robinson S, Ring L, Oxborough D, Harkness A, Bennett S, Rana B, et al. The assessment of left ventricular diastolic function: Guidance and recommendations from the British Society of Echocardiography. Echo Research and Practice. 2024;**11**(1):16

[55] Pelliccia A, Maron BJ, De Luca R, Di Paolo FM, Spataro A, Culasso F. Remodeling of left ventricular hypertrophy in elite athletes after long-term deconditioning. Circulation. 2002;**105**(8):944-949

[56] Pelliccia A, Culasso F, Di Paolo FM, Maron BJ. Physiologic left ventricular cavity dilatation in elite athletes. Annals of Internal Medicine. 1999;**130**(1):23-31

[57] Kapila R, Mahajan RP. Diastolic dysfunction. Continuing Education in Anaesthesia Critical Care & Pain. 2009;**9**(1):29-33

[58] White FC, Bloor CM, McKirnan MD, Carroll SM. Exercise training in swine promotes growth of arteriolar bed and capillary angiogenesis in heart. Journal of Applied Physiology (1985). 1998;**85**(3):1160-1168

[59] Hotta K, Chen B, Behnke BJ, Ghosh P, Stabley JN, Bramy JA, et al. Exercise training reverses age-induced diastolic dysfunction and restores coronary microvascular function. The Journal of Physiology. 2017;**595**(12):3703-3719

[60] Simpson RE, Phillis JW. Adenosine in exercise adaptation. British Journal of Sports Medicine. 1992;**26**(1):54-58

[61] Francis M, Waldrup JR, Qian X, Solodushko V, Meriwether J, Taylor MS. Functional tuning of intrinsic endothelial Ca^{2+} dynamics in swine coronary arteries. Circulation Research. 2016;**118**(7):1078-1090

[62] Ray CJ, Marshall JM. The cellular mechanisms by which adenosine evokes

release of nitric oxide from rat aortic endothelium. The Journal of Physiology. 2006;**570**(Pt 1):85-96

[63] Headrick JP, Ashton KJ, Rose'meyer RB, Peart JN. Cardiovascular adenosine receptors: Expression, actions and interactions. Pharmacology & Therapeutics. 2013;**140**(1):92-111

[64] Loffler M, Morote-Garcia JC, Eltzschig SA, Coe IR, Eltzschig HK. Physiological roles of vascular nucleoside transporters. Arteriosclerosis, Thrombosis, and Vascular Biology. 2007;**27**(5):1004-1013

[65] Tune JD, Richmond KN, Gorman MW, Olsson RA, Feigl EO. Adenosine is not responsible for local metabolic control of coronary blood flow in dogs during exercise. American Journal of Physiology. Heart and Circulatory Physiology. 2000;**278**(1):H74-H84

[66] Sato A, Terata K, Miura H, Toyama K, Loberiza FR Jr, Hatoum OA, et al. Mechanism of vasodilation to adenosine in coronary arterioles from patients with heart disease. American Journal of Physiology. Heart and Circulatory Physiology. 2005;**288**(4):H1633-H1640

[67] Duncker DJ, van Zon NS, Ishibashi Y, Bache RJ. Role of K+ ATP channels and adenosine in the regulation of coronary blood flow during exercise with normal and restricted coronary blood flow. The Journal of Clinical Investigation. 1996;**97**(4):996-1009

[68] Duncker DJ, van Zon NS, Pavek TJ, Herrlinger SK, Bache RJ. Endogenous adenosine mediates coronary vasodilation during exercise after K(ATP)+ channel blockade. The Journal of Clinical Investigation. 1995;**95**(1):285-295

[69] Barron JT, Gu L. Energetic effects of adenosine on vascular smooth muscle. American Journal of Physiology. Heart and Circulatory Physiology. 2000;**278**(1):H26-H32

[70] Roque FR, Soci UP, De Angelis K, Coelho MA, Furstenau CR, Vassallo DV, et al. Moderate exercise training promotes adaptations in coronary blood flow and adenosine production in normotensive rats. Clinics (São Paulo, Brazil). 2011;**66**(12):2105-2111

[71] Yada T, Shimokawa H, Hiramatsu O, Shinozaki Y, Mori H, Goto M, et al. Important role of endogenous hydrogen peroxide in pacing-induced metabolic coronary vasodilation in dogs in vivo. Journal of the American College of Cardiology. 2007;**50**(13):1272-1278

[72] Edelmann F, Gelbrich G, Dungen HD, Frohling S, Wachter R, Stahrenberg R, et al. Exercise training improves exercise capacity and diastolic function in patients with heart failure with preserved ejection fraction: Results of the ex-DHF (exercise training in diastolic heart failure) pilot study. Journal of the American College of Cardiology. 2011;**58**(17):1780-1791

[73] Chaveles I, Papazachou O, Shamari MA, Delis D, Ntalianis A, Panagopoulou N, et al. Effects of exercise training on diastolic and systolic dysfunction in patients with chronic heart failure. World Journal of Cardiology. 2021;**13**(9):514-525

Chapter 2

Hemodynamic Study on Exercise-Based Cardiovascular Rehabilitation and Health Promotion

Yahui Zhang, Xiaodong Zhang, Chaoyang Wang and Kai Liu

Abstract

From the perspective of cardiac rehabilitation and health promotion, this chapter mainly investigates the cardiovascular function response during exercise rehabilitation based on hemodynamic analysis and multimodal physiological signal processing. The first part includes the definitions of cardiac rehabilitation and health promotion, as well as the methods and approaches of exercise rehabilitation. The second part presents the principle of methods, including hemodynamics, blood flow and pulse wave. The third, fourth, and fifth parts respectively relied on hemodynamic analysis and multimodal physiological indicators to study the effects of different exercise modes on cardiovascular disease, the response of passive exercise-Enhanced External Counterpulsation (EECP) to cardiovascular function, and to identify the optimal blood flow indicators for personalized treatment. This chapter aims to provide new research ideas for sports rehabilitation and sports physiology research.

Keywords: cardiac rehabilitation, exercise modality, hemodynamics, enhanced external counterpulsation, cardiovascular disease

1. Introduction

1.1 Definition of cardiovascular rehabilitation

The World Health Organization (WHO) defines cardiac rehabilitation as a comprehensive support system for patients with cardiovascular disease (CVD), encompassing physical, psychological, and social dimensions, to gradually restore patients' social functionality following illness. The primary target population includes individuals with coronary artery disease (CAD), such as those with angina pectoris, myocardial infarction, and recipients of cardiopulmonary transplantation [1]. In addition, the American Association of Cardiovascular and Pulmonary Rehabilitation (AACVPR) and the American Heart Association (AHA) broadly define cardiac rehabilitation as an integrated, coordinated, and sustainable long-term program. This program includes exercise prescription, CVD risk assessment and stratification, patient education, and behavioral interventions [2].

1.2 Overview of exercise rehabilitation and health promotion

1.2.1 Overview of cardiac rehabilitation

The 2023 position paper by the European Society of Cardiology (ESC) states that exercise-based rehabilitation is a structured and individualized intervention strategy that employs prescribed physical activity to restore functional capacity, regulate cardiovascular risk, and improve the quality of life in patients with cardiovascular or metabolic diseases [3]. According to the Chinese Guidelines for Cardiac Rehabilitation and Secondary Prevention 2021, "exercise rehabilitation" is defined as a comprehensive intervention based on medical evaluation and exercise risk assessment, involving aerobic training, resistance training, flexibility exercises, and neuromuscular conditioning, to improve cardiopulmonary function and reduce the risk of recurrent cardiovascular events [4]. Evidence-based medicine has firmly established exercise rehabilitation as the cornerstone of cardiac rehabilitation. A systematic review demonstrated that regular physical activity reduces all-cause mortality by 13% and the risk of rehospitalization due to heart failure by 28%, while significantly improving peak oxygen uptake (VO_2 peak) and quality of life [5]. Furthermore, findings from the national Heart Failure Center Registry Study in China confirmed a 25% reduction in one-year mortality among patients who underwent exercise rehabilitation [6].

1.2.2 Overview of health promotion

Health promotion is classically defined by the World Health Organization (WHO) in the 1986 Ottawa Charter as "the process of enabling people to increase control over, and to improve, their health." This process involves integrating public health policy, creating supportive environments, promoting community action, developing personal skills, and reorienting health services to make healthy choices the easy choices [7]. As a core strategy in both primary and secondary prevention of CVD, health promotion systematically reduces exposure to risk factors by integrating individual behavioral interventions, community mobilization, and supportive policy environments. One notable example is Finland's "North Karelia Project," which implemented interventions such as salt reduction, smoking cessation, promotion of low-fat diets, and community-based physical activity. Over 25 years, the average population systolic blood pressure declined by 11 mmHg, and coronary heart disease mortality decreased by 73%, demonstrating the long-term effectiveness of comprehensive health promotion strategies in reducing CVD risk at the population level [8].

1.3 Overview of exercise rehabilitation and its modality

1.3.1 Exercise modalities in cardiac rehabilitation

As defined, cardiac rehabilitation involves a comprehensive intervention strategy targeting CVD patients, encompassing both physiological and psychological dimensions [9]. Among these, exercise serves as the core component of cardiac rehabilitation. Clinically, two main exercise modalities are widely recommended by international guidelines tailored to specific CVD conditions. The first is active exercise-based rehabilitation, which emphasizes cardiopulmonary training. This includes aerobic exercise, cycle ergometry, and cardiopulmonary exercise testing (CPET), all of which are commonly implemented in clinical settings [1, 10]. The second is referred to in international expert consensus as passive exercise, namely Enhanced External Counterpulsation (EECP), a non-invasive mechanical intervention. EECP has been widely endorsed by both domestic and international guidelines for the management of angina pectoris and coronary artery disease [11]. Both approaches are non-invasive and drug-free modalities that play essential roles in the prevention and treatment of cardiovascular diseases.

1.3.2 Active exercise-based rehabilitation

Cardiac rehabilitation is a coordinated, multidisciplinary intervention designed to optimize a cardiovascular patient's physical, psychological, and social functioning, in addition to stabilizing, slowing, or even reversing the progression of the underlying atherosclerotic processes, thereby reducing morbidity and mortality [10]. The program primarily consists of baseline functional assessment, risk stratification, and the formulation of individualized rehabilitation protocols.

Baseline functional assessment represents a critical component of CR and typically involves evaluation of cardiopulmonary endurance, cardiac structure and function, clinical symptoms and signs, activities of daily living, and psychological status [11].

Risk assessment is another key step in CR. According to the American College of Sports Medicine (ACSM) guidelines, in addition to exercise testing results, other comorbidities—such as type 1 diabetes, morbid obesity, severe pulmonary disease, and neurological disorders—should also be taken into account. Based on the findings of baseline functional assessment and risk stratification, the multidisciplinary healthcare team can tailor individualized rehabilitation plans for each patient [12].

According to the "Core Components of Cardiac Rehabilitation Programs: 2024 Update" jointly released by the American Heart Association (AHA) and the American Association of Cardiovascular and Pulmonary Rehabilitation (AACVPR), exercise training in CR primarily includes aerobic and resistance training. Aerobic exercise is recommended ≥5 times per week, lasting 30–60 minutes per session, with intensity prescribed according to heart rate reserve (HRR) or VO_2 reserve, typically at 40–80% of peak VO_2, which corresponds to 60–90% of peak heart rate [12]. Common modalities include walking, cycling, and swimming. Resistance training is recommended 2–3 times per week, starting at low intensity with light-to-moderate loads, performing 8–15 repetitions per set, and progressively increasing the workload to enhance weight-bearing capacity and skeletal muscle strength. Furthermore, warm-up and cool-down activities are essential before and after exercise sessions to raise body temperature, improve joint flexibility, lower heart rate, and reduce muscle tension [11].

1.3.3 Passive exercise-based rehabilitation: Enhanced external counterpulsation (EECP)

EECP is a non-invasive circulatory support device utilized as a passive adjunctive therapy for the treatment of ischemic cardiovascular conditions. In the 1970s, Professor Zhensheng Zheng and his research team at Sun Yat-sen University successfully developed a sequential limb pneumatic compression system with independent intellectual property rights, which became known as EECP [13]. The device was first clinically applied in 1982 for the treatment of CAD and angina pectoris, and in 1992, it received FDA approval in the United States for use in conditions including stable and unstable angina, acute myocardial infarction, and cardiogenic shock [14]. In 2013, the ESC incorporated EECP into its clinical practice guidelines for the management of stable coronary artery disease, assigning it a Class IIa recommendation [15].

The working principle of EECP involves the identification of the R wave on the electrocardiogram (ECG) to synchronize pneumatic inflation. Air cuffs placed on the calves, thighs, and buttocks inflate sequentially from distal to proximal during diastole, compressing the lower body arteries and augmenting retrograde blood flow toward the upper body. This process enhances perfusion of vital organs, such as the heart and brain. Simultaneously, venous compression increases venous return to the right heart, thereby improving preload. During systole, all three cuffs deflate rapidly, resulting in a reduction in afterload [16]. Recent studies have shown that EECP therapy can alleviate anginal symptoms, improve endothelial function, and enhance myocardial perfusion, making it a non-invasive and innovative approach for the prevention and management of coronary artery disease [17].

2. Basic principles of hemodynamics

Hemodynamics is the physical study of flowing blood and of all the solid structures (such as arteries) through which it flows. At a fundamental level, the study of hemodynamics is concerned with the distribution of pressures and flows in the circulatory system [18]. It encompasses parameters such as blood pressure, vascular resistance, blood flow, flow velocity, and the mechanical properties of the arterial walls, as well as the interrelationships among these factors. In clinical practice, hemodynamic parameters are commonly employed to reveal physiological or pathological changes, to assess the response to therapeutic interventions, and to monitor the progression of disease states [19]. Among the key non-invasive, repeatable, and exercise-related diagnostic techniques are Doppler ultrasound flow spectrum analysis, pulse wave analysis, blood pressure and arterial stiffness measurements, and photoplethysmography (PPG). These modalities play essential roles in the functional evaluation of cardiovascular health and its dynamic changes during rehabilitation [20].

2.1 Ultrasonic blood flow spectrum analysis

Doppler ultrasound technology converts frequency shift signals—representing time-varying blood flow velocities—into a visual spectrum plotted in either frequency–amplitude or velocity–time coordinates. This modality is widely used for evaluating key hemodynamic parameters, including peak velocity, vessel diameter, blood flow volume, and resistance index [21]. Although the blood flow spectrum is conventionally a two-dimensional image, several studies have explored advanced signal and image processing techniques to extract blood velocity waveforms. These methods often involve region of interest (ROI) segmentation, binarization, morphological closing operations, and Sobel edge detection to delineate the spectral envelope. Once the blood flow velocity waveform is obtained, it can be analyzed to extract multiple types of features: Waveform morphology and time-domain features.

Frequency-domain features via the Fourier transform, including power spectral density, sub-band energy analysis, and transfer function characteristics. These quantitative descriptors offer detailed insights into vascular function and flow dynamics, and they are increasingly used in both clinical assessment and research on cardiovascular rehabilitation [22, 23].

2.2 Blood pressure and arterial stiffness

Studies have shown that continuous acquisition of pulse wave signals is essential for the detection of blood pressure and arterial stiffness [24]. By analyzing pulse waveforms, it is possible to construct models for real-time, continuous blood pressure monitoring, which allows for the assessment of systolic blood pressure (SBP), diastolic blood pressure (DBP), mean arterial pressure (MAP), as well as indicators of arterial stiffness [25]. One such indicator is the Augmentation Index (AIx), which represents the percentage of central pulse pressure attributed to reflected waves. An elevated AIx indicates earlier return of pulse wave reflections and increased central arterial load, and is positively associated with left ventricular hypertrophy and an increased risk of heart failure. A 10% increase in AIx corresponds to an 8% rise in peak wall shear stress, which accelerates endothelial dysfunction and the progression of atherosclerosis [26]. Another key parameter is Pulse Wave Velocity (PWV), which measures the speed at which the pulse wave propagates through the arterial tree following ventricular ejection. The most commonly used index is the carotid–femoral PWV (cf-PWV). PWV is linearly correlated with arterial stiffness and serves as an independent predictor of cardiovascular events. Specifically, for every 1 m/s increase in cf-PWV, the risk of cardiovascular events rises by approximately 15% [27].

2.3 Photoplethysmography (PPG) analysis

PPG is a simple, non-invasive optical measurement technique used to monitor changes in blood volume within the microvascular bed of peripheral tissues [20, 28] At present, this technology has been widely applied in the measurement of blood pressure and hemodynamic parameters [29], the prediction of cardiovascular diseases [30], the assessment of chronic conditions, and the early warning of stroke risk [31]. The second derivative of the PPG signal (SDPPG) has been widely adopted as a simple and reliable indicator of elevated arterial pressure in clinical research [32]. SDPPG reflects not only the ascending aortic systolic pressure wave but also serves as a biomarker of vascular aging [32–34]. Moreover, SDPPG is closely associated with several established cardiovascular risk indicators [35–37].

2.3.1 Extraction and applications of the second derivative of PPG

Direct extraction of the second derivative from raw PPG waveforms often fails to accurately identify the key morphological features—namely, the a, b, c, d, and e inflection points. To address this limitation, the Fourier fitting method is commonly employed to compute and extract these characteristic points more precisely. This SDPPG fitting approach aims to achieve a reliable and accurate detection of the waveform's critical second-derivative features [38].

The SDPPG waveform contains five characteristic points: Point a: the first positive peak in the cycle, closely associated with the onset of the systolic upstroke in the original PPG signal; Point b: the following negative trough, corresponding to the maximum of the systolic phase in the PPG signal; Points c, d, and e: inflection points related to changes in the slope of the diastolic wave (See **Figure 1**). Based on multi-physiological signal acquisition, this section calculates and analyzes several derived hemodynamic indices, including: b/a: the amplitude ratio of point b to a in the SDPPG; e/a, c/a, and d/a: the amplitude ratios of points e, c, and d to a, respectively; $(b - c - d - e)/a$, also referred to as the Aging Index (AGI). In conditions where

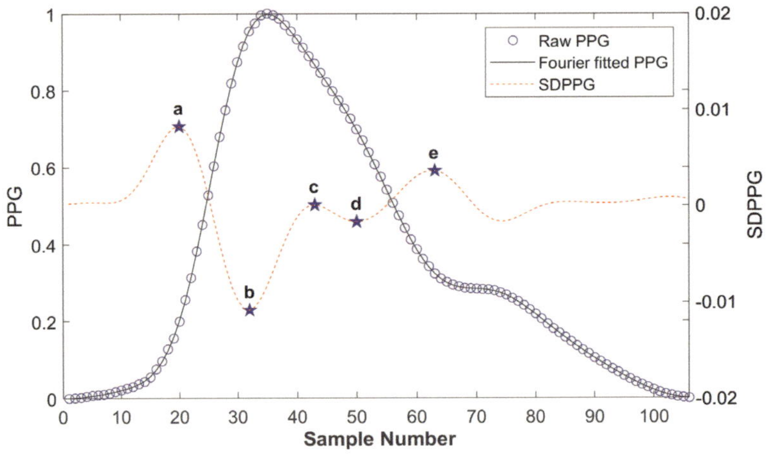

Figure 1.
Typical PPG and its second derivative in a cardiac cycle based on Fourier fitting from a healthy subject at rest. (The black solid line is the raw PPG, and the open circles are the Fourier fitted data. The asterisk is the feature point of SDPPG [39]. Source: *https://www.frontiersin.org/journals/physiology/articles/10.3389/fphys.2018.01590/full.*

points b and c are absent (e.g., during intense physical activity), AGI is alternatively calculated as (b–e)/a. These amplitude ratios—b/a, c/a, d/a, e/a, and (b − c − d − e)/a —are extracted from the SDPPG waveform and serve as quantitative markers of systolic and diastolic vascular function. Second derivative photoplethysmography (SDPPG), through its characteristic waveform components (a, b, c, d, and e waves), provides valuable information for the assessment of cardiovascular status. Among these, the b/a ratio is a key index for evaluating arterial stiffness, as it increases with worsening stiffness [40]. In addition, the c/a, d/a, and e/a ratios can be applied to assess arterial health, whereas the (b − c − d − e)/a or (b − e)/a ratios are useful for evaluating vascular aging and atherosclerosis. Owing to its high sensitivity and non-invasive nature, SDPPG enables real-time monitoring of cardiovascular status and offers valuable support for the early diagnosis and management of cardiovascular disease [39, 41].

2.3.2 Extraction and application of PPG morphological features

The morphological contour of the PPG signal holds significant value for cardiovascular risk assessment [20]. To investigate hemodynamic responses before, during, and after exercise, key morphological features of the PPG waveform were extracted, as illustrated in **Figure 2**.

Based on the extracted features from the PPG waveform, the following indices were calculated to reflect hemodynamic changes:

1. Stiffness Index (SI)

   Assuming that the pulse wave path length is proportional to body height (H), the SI is defined as: SI (m/s) = H/ΔTBVP, where ΔTBVP is the time difference between the systolic and diastolic peaks of the PPG waveform. SI is regarded as an indicator of pulse contour characteristics related to blood volume and is primarily determined by the pulse wave velocity in the aorta and large arteries [38].

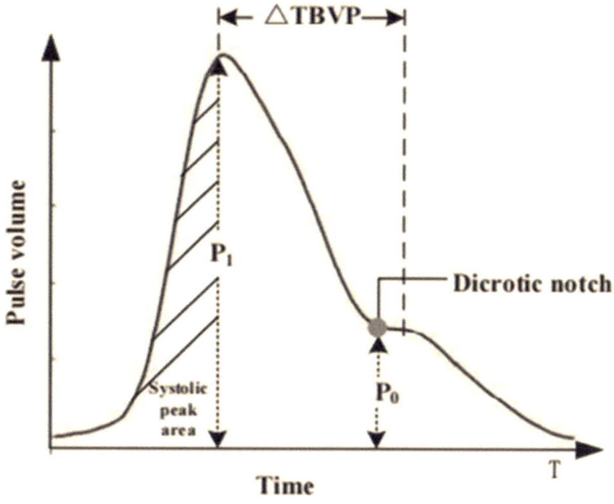

Figure 2.
Morphological characteristics extraction of the PPG signal.

2. P_0/P_1

This ratio quantifies the volume pulse during systole. P_0 represents the amplitude of the PPG signal at the dicrotic notch, while P_1 represents the amplitude at the systolic peak. The ratio P_0/P_1 is calculated as the amplitude from the onset point to the notch (valley) divided by the amplitude from the foot point to the systolic peak [38].

3. S_area – Area Under the Systolic Peak

The S_area is defined as the area under the systolic portion of the PPG waveform, measured from the waveform onset to the systolic peak [38].

4. ΔTBVP / T Ratio

This index represents the time delay between the systolic and diastolic peaks. T is the time duration of one complete PPG cycle. The PPG waveform often shows an early systolic peak followed shortly by a second peak or inflection point during early diastole. The time interval between these two points, denoted as ΔTBVP, serves as a non-invasive measure of the time required for pulse wave reflection, commonly used to evaluate arterial stiffness, particularly in the subclavian artery [38].

5. K-Value

The K-value is a simplified quantitative index proposed by Professor Zhichang Luo at Beijing University of Technology, based on the relationship between vascular resistance, arterial elasticity, and changes in the area under the PPG waveform. It is defined as:

$$K = \frac{P_m - P_d}{P_s - P_d} \tag{1}$$

Where: P_m is the mean arterial pressure, P_d is the diastolic pressure P_s is the systolic pressure. As vascular resistance increases—for example, with aging or arteriosclerosis—the PPG waveform changes from a sharp, steep profile to a broader, dome-shaped pattern, and the K-value increases accordingly, typically ranging between 0.35 and 0.5. Morphological analysis of photoplethysmography (PPG) signals provides a novel perspective for understanding cardiovascular physiology and pathophysiology. Morphological features include signal smoothness, the number of local extrema, entropy, and root mean square (RMS), all of which reflect dynamic changes in the microcirculation. For example, smoothness and the number of local extrema describe the jaggedness of the signal, whereas entropy reflects its complexity. In one study, morphological analysis of PPG signals revealed that photobiomodulation (PBM) significantly increased signal amplitude and reduced jaggedness, indicating a beneficial effect of PBM on microcirculatory function [42].

3. Immediate effects of cardiopulmonary exercise testing on cardiovascular health

Hypertension is the most common cause of cardiovascular morbidity and mortality, and one of the primary modifiable risk factors for cardiovascular disease. It is closely associated with the development of atherosclerosis and cerebrovascular diseases [43, 44]. Although the progression of CVD is strongly linked to structural and functional changes in the arterial system, the presence of various risk factors significantly accelerates its course, among which hypertension is considered one of the most critical [45]. Given the multifactorial nature and complexity of hypertension, its underlying pathophysiological mechanisms require further investigation. CPET is regarded as the gold standard for the comprehensive assessment of exercise response and the diagnosis of cardiopulmonary functional capacity [43, 46]. Several studies have reported that CPET can be used to predict and evaluate cardiovascular risk [35, 43]. Analyzing cardiovascular characteristics during CPET may provide valuable insights into arterial stiffness and help in assessing overall cardiovascular risk and vascular dysfunction.

3.1 Second derivative variation of PPG

Studies have shown that before CPET, there were no significant differences between the untreated hypertension subjects (UHS) and healthy subjects (HS) in terms of b/a, d/a, and AGI [39]. However, following CPET, b/a and AGI were significantly higher in the UHS group compared to the HS group, whereas d/a and c/a were significantly lower in the UHS than in the HS. In contrast, e/a was significantly lower in UHS before CPET, but no significant intergroup difference was observed after the test. Furthermore, compared with pre-CPET values, both UHS and HS groups exhibited a significant increase in AGI during exercise, with UHS demonstrating a markedly higher AGI post-CPET. Notably, no significant difference in c/a and d/a was found between the two groups during CPET [39]. Differences in exercise responses revealed disparities in cardiopulmonary function between untreated hypertensive subjects (UHS) and healthy subjects (HS). These differences not only underscore the elevated cardiovascular (CV) risk in UHS but also serve as predictors of future arterial stiffening. Furthermore, compared with the pre-CPET (cardiopulmonary exercise testing) state, significant differences were observed between the two groups during

CPET in terms of arterial compliance index (AGI), autonomic nervous system function, and respiratory activity. In summary, this study demonstrates that exercise response is an effective approach to characterize cardiopulmonary functional differences between UHS and HS, while also providing valuable predictive and diagnostic information for cardiovascular disease (CVD) [39].

In this study, no significant differences in b/a, d/a, or AGI were observed between the two groups before CPET. However, post-exercise measurements revealed marked differences, suggesting that physical exertion may serve as an effective physiological stressor to explore cardiovascular functional differences between healthy individuals and those with untreated hypertension [39].

Large-cohort studies have indicated that lower b/a, higher d/a, and higher AGI reflect increased arterial stiffness, serving as markers of arteriosclerosis [32]. Moreover, changes in these three parameters are considered reliable indicators of the vascular pathophysiology affecting both large central arteries and peripheral arteries in hypertensive patients [47]. By contrast, some reports have suggested that these parameters may have limited sensitivity in detecting macrovascular pathophysiological changes in patients with target organ damage [48], further implying that SDPPG indices may be more closely associated with microvascular changes than with large arterial alterations [48].

During exercise, c/a and d/a were not detected in either group. Previous studies have shown that a decrease in c/a is associated with impaired baroreflex sensitivity and reduced cardiac parasympathetic tone [49]. In addition, c/a has been linked to hypertension, diabetes, hyperlipidemia, and elevated total cholesterol levels [49]. Several studies have also reported that reductions in these parameters are related to increased arterial stiffness and aging [47, 50].

3.2 Evaluation of blood pressure and arterial stiffness changes before, during, and after CPET using PPG morphological features

Statistical analyses of PPG morphological features were performed to evaluate hemodynamic changes across the CPET timeline (pre-, intra-, and post-exercise) [39]. The results revealed distinct variations in several PPG-derived indices, including the SI, P_0/P_1 ratio, S_area (area under the systolic peak), ΔTBVP/T ratio, and the K-value [38]. During CPET, both the UHS (untreated hypertension subjects) and HS (healthy subjects) groups showed a significant decrease in P_0/P_1 and S_area compared to their pre-exercise values. In contrast, the ΔTBVP/T ratio and K-value increased significantly during exercise in both groups. For UHS, significant changes in ΔTBVP/T were observed not only between pre- and intra-exercise, but also between intra- and post-exercise, as well as pre- and post-exercise. However, in the HS group, no significant change in ΔTBVP/T was observed across the exercise phases. In addition, SI showed significant differences in the HS group during and after CPET, compared to pre-exercise values. Notably, P_0/P_1 and ΔTBVP/T ratio differed significantly between UHS and HS before exercise, but no significant intergroup difference was detected during or after CPET. The S_area parameter did not differ significantly pre-CPET but became significantly different post-exercise [38].

To assess continuous hemodynamic changes across the entire CPET process, the study further analyzed several physiological parameters derived from waveform features, including Pulse Transit Time (PTT), Blood Pressure (BP), and Heart Rate Variability (HRV) indices—specifically the high-frequency (HF) and low-frequency

(LF) components. The temporal trends of these parameters across pre-, intra-, and post-exercise phases were compared [38].

A significant intergroup difference was found in the rate of change of LF during exercise ($p = 0.000$), with UHS showing a distinct pattern compared to HS. While the rate of blood pressure (BP) change did not differ significantly between groups, both showed notable BP elevation during exercise. It is hypothesized that the mechanisms of BP elevation differ between groups: in HS, the increase may reflect physiological sympathetic activation, whereas in UHS, it could be a compensatory response due to elevated baseline BP and an urgent need to meet oxygen demand under increased workload. This hypothesis warrants further validation through animal experiments [39].

In summary, the observed differences in PPG morphological features, BP, PTT, and HRV indices between hypertensive and healthy individuals at various stages of exercise provide valuable insights into the cardiovascular functional dynamics during rehabilitation. These findings offer theoretical support for clinical rehabilitation assessment and personalized treatment planning.

4. The impact of different exercise modes on Hemodynamics of different cardiovascular diseases

According to the most recent epidemiological statistics, an estimated 19.41 million deaths worldwide in 2021 were attributable to cardiovascular disease, corresponding to an age-standardized mortality rate of 235.18 per 100,000 population. The global prevalence of cardiovascular disease reached approximately 612.06 million cases, with an age-standardized prevalence rate of 7178.73 per 100,000 population [51]. Among all regions, Central Asia and Eastern Europe reported the highest mortality rates, whereas the lowest rates were observed in high-income Asia-Pacific countries and Australia [52]. Physical inactivity has been identified as the fourth leading risk factor for global mortality, contributing to approximately 69.3 million disability-adjusted life years (DALYs) in 2010 [53, 54]. Engaging in regular physical activity is widely regarded as a major contributor to both the prevention and rehabilitation of CVD [55, 56]. Exercise-based cardiac rehabilitation, including aerobic endurance training, dynamic resistance training, and combined modalities, has been implemented to improve cardiovascular health in patients with CVD [56]. Hemodynamics is the biophysical study of circulating blood and the luminal structures through which it flows, such as arteries and the heart. It encompasses blood pressure, vascular resistance, blood flow, flow velocity, and the physical properties of arterial walls, as well as the interrelationships among these parameters. However, the differential effects of various exercise modalities on cardiovascular function and hemodynamic parameters in patients with different types of CVD remain unclear. To address this gap in knowledge, a meta-analysis and regression study was conducted to evaluate the impact of specific exercise interventions on cardiovascular and hemodynamic outcomes across different CVD populations [57].

4.1 Aerobic exercise

4.1.1 Effects of aerobic exercise on central hemodynamic variables

Aortic Systolic Pressure (ASP) represents the peak pressure in the ascending aorta during the ventricular ejection phase, reflecting the interaction between left ventricular stroke volume, the rate of ejection, and the buffering capacity (compliance) of the aorta

[58]. Based on a fixed-effects model, aerobic exercise was found to significantly improve ASP (See **Figure 3**). Aortic Diastolic Pressure (ADP) is the minimum pressure reached in the aorta at the end of the diastole, immediately before the next ventricular contraction. It is primarily determined by the systemic vascular resistance and the duration of the diastolic decay. The analysis revealed a significant reduction in ADP following aerobic training (See **Figure 4**). The augmentation index (AIx) is defined as the ratio of augmentation pressure to pulse pressure and is considered a surrogate measure of arterial stiffness and wave reflection intensity [24]. Among patients with cardiovascular disease, no significant change in AIx was observed following aerobic exercise (See **Figure 5**). Meta-regression analysis further demonstrated that AIx was not significantly affected by age, sex, type of disease, or exercise duration. In this meta-analysis, 10 trials evaluating aerobic exercise reported measurements of AIx, but only 4 of these studies (n = 152) included data on heart rate–adjusted AIx. Results indicated no significant changes in heart rate–adjusted AIx following aerobic training. Notably, compared with brachial blood pressure, both aerobic and resistance exercise induce significant improvements in central blood pressure, which is considered a stronger predictor of target organ damage, as well as in cardiovascular morbidity and mortality among patients with cardiovascular disease [59, 60]. Specifically, studies on the effects of aerobic exercise on augmentation index (AIx) have demonstrated that AIx is significantly reduced either after 24 weeks of aerobic training or in patients aged 50–60 years. Interestingly, these changes appear to be independent of sex, disease status, and heart rate. Nevertheless, several reports have suggested that AIx may still be influenced by age and disease, since arterial reservoir pressure increases rapidly with advancing age and pathological conditions [61, 62]. Furthermore, AIx may also be modulated by additional hemodynamic and exercise-related factors, including left ventricular afterload, exercise intensity, frequency, and duration, central wave reflection, forward wave generation, and vascular impedance [62–65]. Collectively, these findings highlight that AIx is determined not only by pulse wave reflection but also by the compliance of elastic arteries [66].

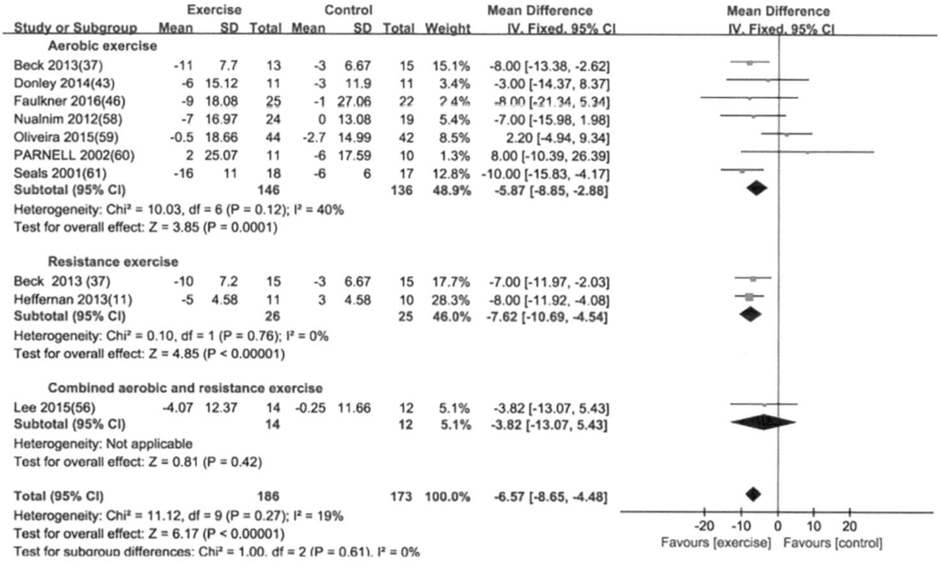

Figure 3.
Forest plot of the change in ASP in the exercise and control groups [57]. (Source: https://journals.plos.org/plosone/article?id=10.1371/journal.pone.0200829).

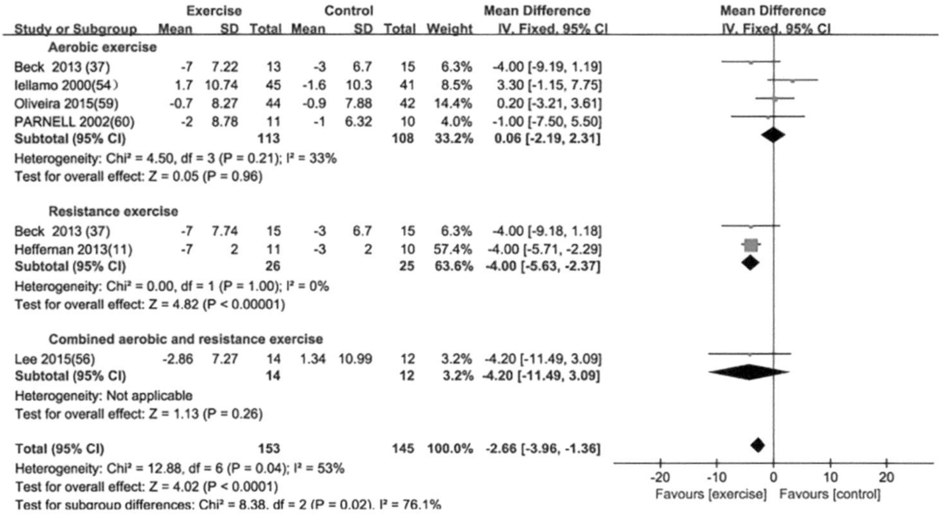

Figure 4.
Forest plot of the change in ADP in the exercise and control groups [57]. (Source: https://journals.plos.org/plosone/article?id=10.1371/journal.pone.0200829).

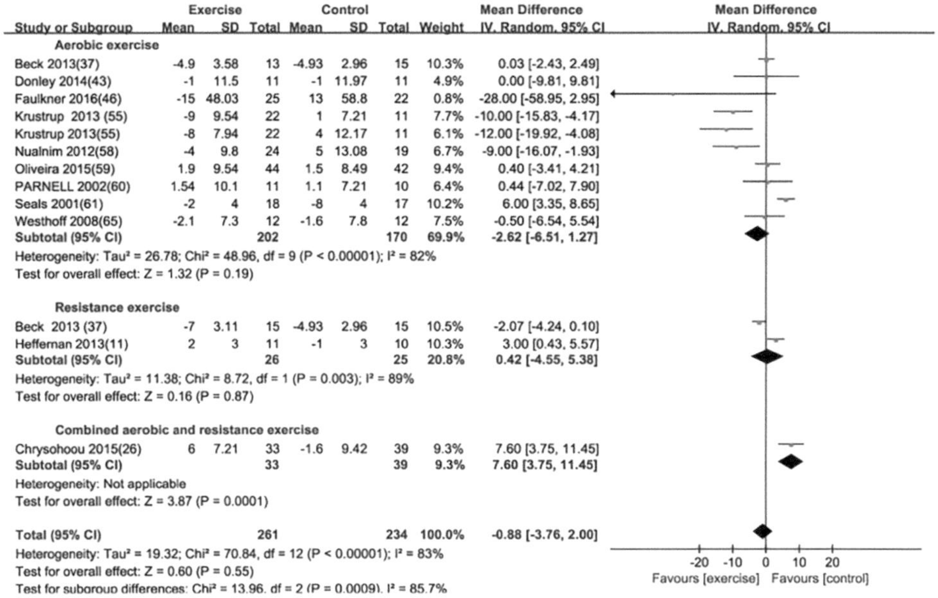

Figure 5.
Forest plot of the change in central AIX in the exercise and control groups [57]. (Source: https://journals.plos.org/plosone/article?id=10.1371/journal.pone.0200829).

4.1.2 Effects of aerobic exercise on central arterial stiffness

Central arterial stiffness refers to the pathological condition characterized by reduced elasticity and increased rigidity of major central arteries such as the aorta and carotid arteries. A stiffening of the large elastic arteries leads to a loss of the buffering

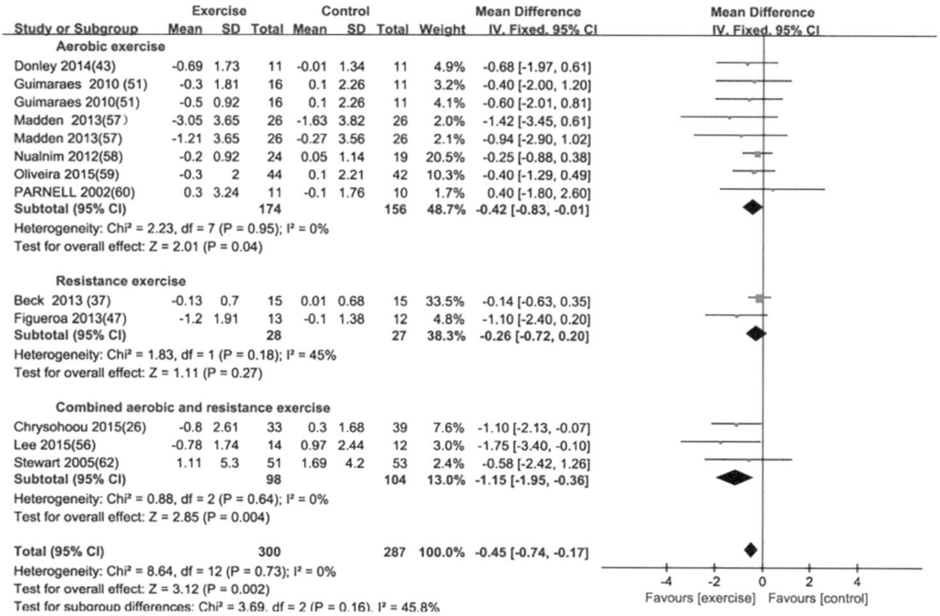

Figure 6.
Forest plot of the change in carotid-femoral pulse wave velocity (cf-PWV) in the exercise and control groups [57]. (Source: https://journals.plos.org/plosone/article?id=10.1371/journal.pone.0200829).

capacity of the vasculature, which increases the transmission of pulsatile energy to the microcirculation [24]. Carotid–femoral pulse wave velocity (cf-PWV) is considered the gold standard for evaluating central arterial stiffness. It measures the speed at which the pulse wave travels between the carotid and femoral arteries [24]. Among patients with CVD, aerobic exercise was found to significantly reduce cf-PWV, indicating a beneficial effect on central arterial stiffness (See **Figure 6**). Studies have shown that aerobic exercise reduces cf-PWV in patients with cardiovascular disease as well as in the general adult population [64, 67, 68]. The improvement in cf-PWV through aerobic exercise may be attributed to several mechanisms, including enhanced nitric oxide (NO) bioavailability, increased elastin content in conduit arteries, reduced concentrations of vasoconstrictors, elevated peak oxygen uptake (VO_2 peak), and decreased ASP [64, 69].

4.1.3 Effects of aerobic exercise on cardiac function

The primary role of the heart is to function as a pump, maintaining an adequate cardiac output to meet the metabolic demands of the body. This mechanical performance is the result of a complex interplay between systolic contraction, which ejects blood into the systemic and pulmonary circulations, and diastolic relaxation, which allows the ventricles to fill for the subsequent beat [70]. Two key indicators used to evaluate cardiac function are: Left ventricular ejection fraction (LVEF) – the percentage of blood pumped out of the left ventricle per heartbeat; Cardiac output (CO) – the volume of blood the heart pumps per minute. A total of 7 studies, including 372 patients, demonstrated that aerobic exercise led to a significant improvement in CO (See **Figure 7**) [57]. Furthermore, based on a fixed-effects model, 19 studies involving 843 patients showed that aerobic training significantly increased LVEF (See **Figure 8**)

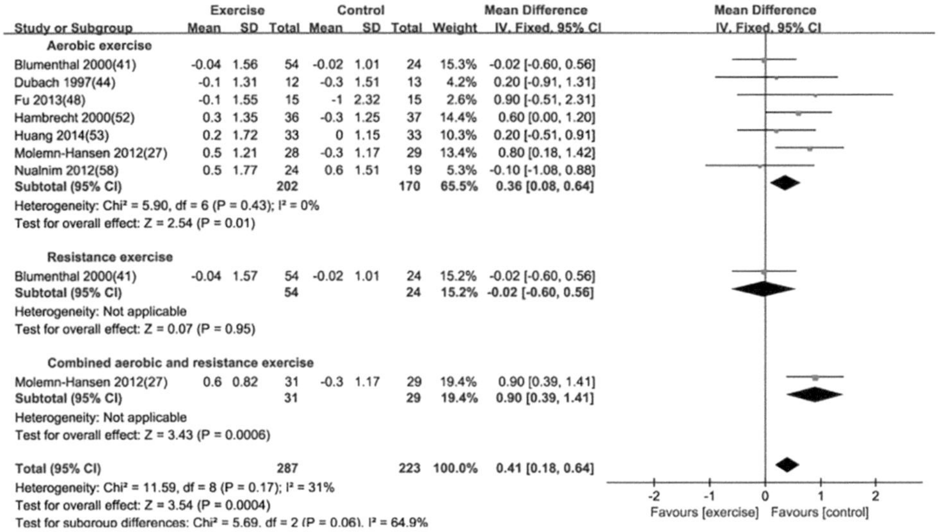

Figure 7.
Forest plot of the change in CO in the exercise and control groups [57]. (Source: https://journals.plos.org/plosone/article?id=10.1371/journal.pone.0200829).

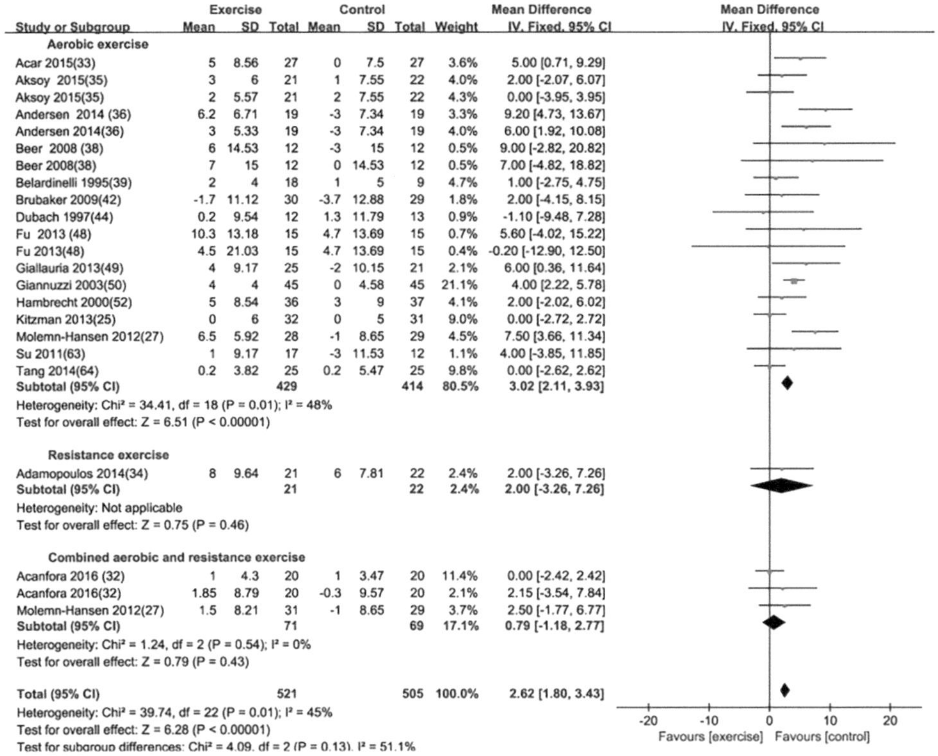

Figure 8.
Forest plot of the change in LVEF in the exercise and control groups [57]. (Source:https://journals.plos.org/plosone/article?id=10.1371/journal.pone.0200829).

[57]. Evidence suggests that aerobic exercise improves ejection fraction (EF) and reverses left ventricular remodeling in patients with heart failure, whereas the additional benefits of combined aerobic and resistance training are less pronounced [71]. In the present study, the effects of aerobic exercise on left ventricular ejection fraction (LVEF) appeared to be age-dependent. Aerobic exercise significantly increased LVEF, likely through its influence on vasoconstrictor neurohormone release, hemodynamic load, peak exercise stroke volume (SV), myocardial contractility, and diastolic filling [71, 72]. The exercise-induced increase in SV has been associated with reduced total peripheral resistance (TPR), driven by sympathetic withdrawal and enhanced parasympathetic tone [73]. In addition, improvements in myocardial contractility further contributed to the augmentation of SV following exercise training [74].

4.2 Resistance exercise

Resistance training was found to significantly improve ASP (See **Figure 3**). It also resulted in a 4 mmHg reduction in ADP, which was statistically significant (See **Figure 4**). One study reported that resistance exercise exerts adverse effects on central blood pressure and arterial compliance [75]. The hypertension induced by resistance training may be primarily associated with increased arterial stiffness [76]. Moreover, greater arterial stiffness has been linked to vascular smooth muscle cell proliferation and pro-inflammatory cytokine activity, thereby contributing to elevations in central blood pressure [77]. However, several alternative mechanisms have been proposed to explain the beneficial effects of resistance training on central blood pressure. Croymans et al. suggested that these benefits may result from improvements in endothelial function and microvascular perfusion [78]. Similarly, Heffernan et al. demonstrated that resistance training significantly improves central blood pressure through its influence on reservoir pressure, which is proportional to the volume of blood stored in the aorta and determined by the interplay between systemic arterial compliance and outflow impedance [63]. In addition, Figueroa and Taaffe reported that these improvements may also be attributed to enhanced vasodilation of peripheral muscular arteries and reductions in peripheral vascular resistance (PVR) [79, 80]. Resistance training has been shown to lower PVR and arteriolar tone, which may alter terminal impedance and facilitate greater blood inflow into the peripheral microvascular bed during diastole (inflow < outflow), ultimately leading to a sustained reduction in reservoir pressure [81].

However, no significant change in AIX was observed in CVD patients following resistance exercise (See **Figure 5**). Studies showed no significant change in carotid–femoral pulse wave velocity cf-PWV after resistance training, indicating no clear effect on central arterial stiffness (See **Figure 6**). Resistance exercise did not lead to significant improvements in CO or LVEF among patients with CVD (See **Figures 8** and **9**). There remains considerable controversy regarding whether resistance training exerts any beneficial effects on left ventricular ejection fraction (LVEF). Some studies have suggested that resistance exercise may increase both systolic and diastolic pressure loads, whereas others have reported that it may augment left ventricular wall stress, subsequently leading to reductions in wall stress, contractile reserve, and preload reserve [72]. In contrast, previous studies have consistently shown that aerobic exercise significantly enhances cardiac output, primarily through improvements in maximal oxygen uptake (VO_2max) related to oxygen delivery, along with reductions in total peripheral resistance, heart rate, and stroke volume, thereby contributing to improved cardiac performance and ventricular filling [83–85]. At present, the impact of resistance training on carotid–femoral pulse wave velocity (cf-PWV) remains

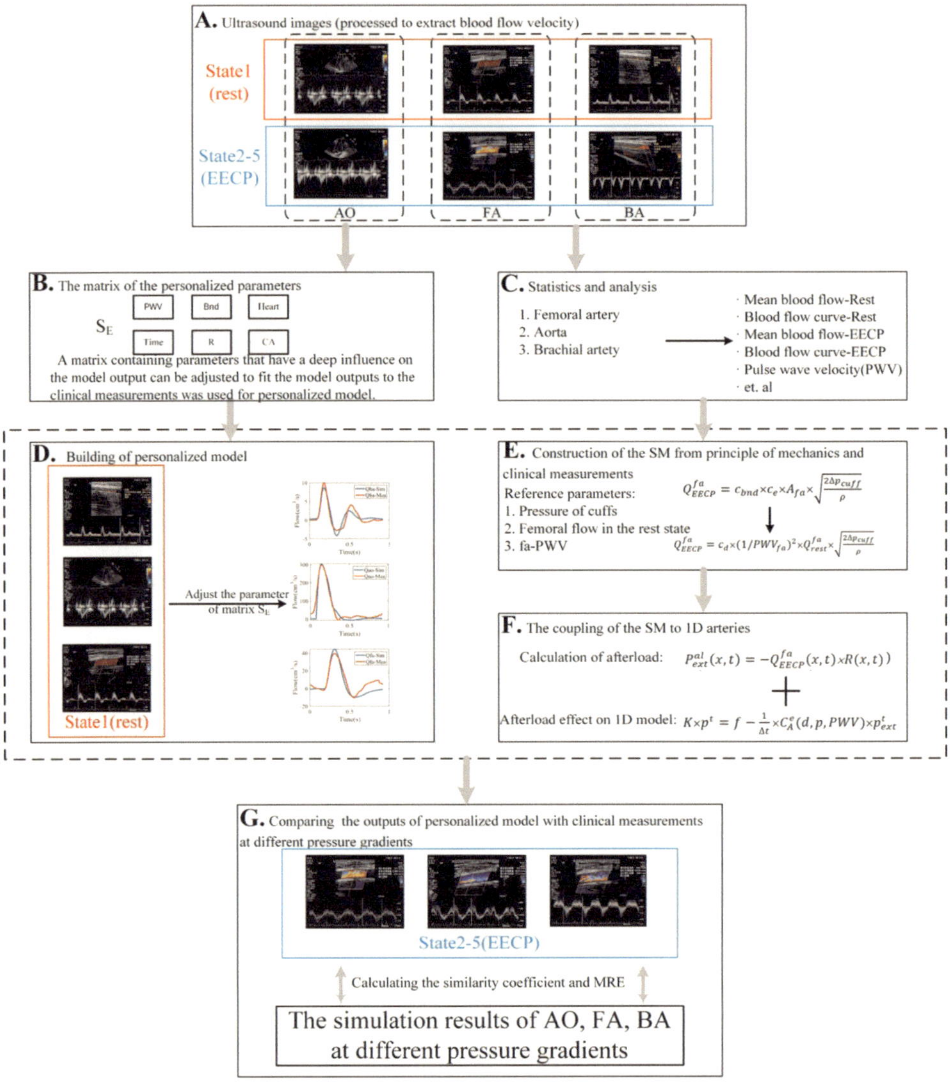

Figure 9.
The flowchart of the approach used in this study [82]. (Source: https://www.sciencedirect.com/science/article/pii/S0021929024001349?via%3Dihub&_cf_chl_tk=iTC8YZpc_NfRgwYcZoZKZmrjC8gR4MVJx9dVzJuBWLs-1773749124-1.0.1.1-8emY4YaEOZxRnj4PANlpHkvsoSgt6Xrk8gxlUbjoF_E).

controversial and appears to be multifactorial [78, 86] Specifically, the effects of resistance exercise may depend not only on exercise intensity and health status but also on arterial compliance and central blood pressure regulation mediated by sympathetic nervous system activity, as well as protein synthesis that modulates muscle mass [67, 86–88].

4.3 Combined exercise

Combined aerobic and resistance training did not significantly improve ASP or ADP (See **Figures 4** and **5**). However, one included study reported a significant increase in Aix following combined exercise in patients with chronic heart failure

(CHF) (See **Figure 5**). Among patients with CVD, combined exercise resulted in a significant reduction in carotid–femoral pulse wave velocity cf-PWV, suggesting improved central arterial stiffness (See **Figure 6**). Combined training significantly increased CO by 0.9 L/min, which was statistically significant in the included studies (See **Figure 7**). However, no significant improvement in LVEF was observed (See **Figure 8**). In one included study [89], no significant differences in ASP or ADP were observed in the combined exercise subgroup. Previous studies have supported the notion that either aerobic or resistance exercise reduces ASP through improvements in vasoactive substances and endothelial function [78–80, 90], and have similarly reported no significant differences in ADP following aerobic exercise [91]. Moreover, a study indicated that when aerobic and resistance exercise are performed within the same training session, combined exercise may exert favorable effects on arterial stiffness [87]. However, these findings contrast with several earlier meta-analyses, which concluded that combined exercise does not significantly affect pulse wave velocity (PWV) [64, 67].

4.4 Summary

Different types of exercise interventions exert varying effects on central hemodynamics, arterial stiffness, and cardiac function in patients with CVD. Both aerobic and resistance exercise significantly reduced ASP. Long-term aerobic training was also associated with a reduction in AIx among CVD patients. Additionally, aerobic and combined exercise were shown to effectively improve central arterial stiffness and cardiac function. The reduction in central blood pressure observed after resistance exercise may be primarily attributed to reduced reservoir pressure or improved microvascular perfusion. In contrast, the improvements in arterial stiffness and cardiac function following aerobic and combined exercise are more likely due to enhancements in cardiorespiratory capacity (as reflected by peak VO_2 related to oxygen delivery and stroke volume) and endothelial function. However, some unexplained heterogeneity remains across the studies included in this review. This is partly due to a lack of high-quality research, particularly regarding the effects of combined exercise on central hemodynamics and arterial stiffness in cardiovascular rehabilitation. In conclusion, these findings hold significant clinical relevance for the rehabilitation of patients with cardiovascular disease. They emphasize the importance of individualized exercise prescriptions, allowing clinicians and rehabilitation specialists to tailor interventions based on specific cardiovascular pathophysiology.

5. Effects of enhanced external counterpulsation on cardiovascular health

EECP, as a passive exercise-based rehabilitation modality, has demonstrated significant potential in the management of cardiovascular and cerebrovascular diseases. The primary physiological effect of EECP lies in its ability to enhance perfusion and improve blood supply to large organs and tissues. Accordingly, most existing research has focused on hemodynamic responses, with ultrasound-based monitoring as the dominant evaluation method. In addition, computational modeling, including simulation and biomechanical analysis, has been used to explore the underlying mechanisms of EECP during the rehabilitation process [92].

Therefore, this chapter focuses on examining the effects and mechanisms of EECP on cardiovascular function by analyzing: Time-domain and frequency-domain characteristics of hemodynamics; Biomechanical parameters derived from 0D–1D hemodynamic models and related simulations. Through these approaches, we aim to provide a mechanistic understanding of EECP's therapeutic role in cardiovascular rehabilitation.

5.1 Acute responses of ultrasound blood flow spectrum characteristics

Studies have shown that long-term EECP therapy significantly improves several hemodynamic parameters, including internal diameter (ID), end-diastolic velocity (EDV), flow rate (FR), resistance index (RI), y2, and peak systolic energy ratio (PSER) at 2.05 Hz. Notably, 35-hour EECP sessions were found to improve hemodynamic function and endothelial function in the common carotid artery, brachial artery, and femoral artery. The beneficial effects of EECP on endothelial function are closely related to the changes in hemodynamics, highlighting the importance of investigating acute hemodynamic responses during EECP as a way to elucidate its mechanistic underpinnings. Moreover, the immediate hemodynamic responses may serve as a predictor of cumulative long-term benefit, providing a reciprocal validation framework [93]. Previous studies have demonstrated that Doppler power spectral analysis improves the early diagnosis of carotid artery disease, enabling the detection of microvascular flow disturbances at subclinical stages [94]. In addition, spectral descriptors of flow velocity waveforms have been shown to better indicate preclinical microvascular abnormalities [95]. Some studies have also reported that low-frequency spectral components contain important information for characterizing hemodynamics [96] and sympathetic nervous system activity [97].

In our previous study [38], we enrolled 94 patients with CAD and 94 matched controls, and analyzed both time-domain and frequency-domain hemodynamic features—including ID, EDV, FR, RI, y2, and PSER (2.05)—before and after EECP treatment. All participants underwent a single 45-minute EECP session. Color Doppler ultrasound (GE Logic E) was used to measure vascular parameters 5 to 25 minutes before and immediately after EECP treatment. Ultrasound assessments of the right and left common carotid arteries (CCA) were standardized to a location approximately 1.5 cm proximal to the bifurcation to measure changes in arterial diameter. The right brachial artery and right femoral artery were measured at anatomically fixed points approximately 5 cm above the antecubital fossa and 2 cm below the inguinal ligament, respectively.

5.1.1 Mean vascular internal diameter (ID)

A significant increase in ID was observed in the brachial and femoral arteries of CAD patients following EECP. However, the left common carotid artery (CCA) showed no significant change during or after EECP in the CAD group. In contrast, the control group exhibited significant ID enlargement in the right CCA and bilateral CCA during and after EECP, while no changes were observed in the brachial or femoral arteries [93].

5.1.2 End-diastolic velocity (EDV)

During EECP and immediately after the 45-minute session, EDV in the CCA and brachial artery decreased significantly in both CAD and control groups. Following EECP, EDV values increased sharply, returning to pre-EECP levels in both arteries

($p < 0.01$), except for the brachial artery in the control group, which did not fully recover. There were no significant changes in femoral artery EDV before or after EECP ($p > 0.05$) [93].

5.1.3 Resistance index (RI)

Although RI in the CCA increased significantly during EECP, it returned quickly to baseline after the session in both CAD and control groups. Post-EECP RI values were substantially lower than those measured before EECP [93].

5.1.4 Flow rate (FR)

After EECP, FR continued to increase in both groups. However, brachial artery FR showed a declining trend, particularly in the control group, while femoral artery FR increased in both groups, with CAD patients exhibiting a more pronounced elevation [93].

5.1.5 Second peak (y_2)

During EECP, the second peak (y_2) in CAD patients increased significantly. However, after EECP, y_2 decreased notably in the left CCA and brachial artery of both groups, with a more prominent reduction observed in the control group [93].

5.1.6 Power spectral energy ratio in the 0–2.05 Hz band (PSER (2.05))

During EECP, PSER (2.05) in both the CCA and brachial artery significantly decreased in both groups. Immediately after EECP, PSER (2.05) increased significantly compared to during EECP ($p < 0.05$). After the 45-minute session, the control group showed a significant increase in PSER (2.05) in both the right CCA (RC) and right femoral artery (RF) compared to baseline; In the CAD group, a significant increase in PSER (2.05) was observed in the right brachial artery (RB) compared to pre-EECP values [93].

5.2 Long-term effects of EECP on hemodynamics

A study was conducted to evaluate the long-term effects of EECP on the hemodynamics of the CCA, brachial artery, and femoral artery in 16 patients with CAD. During treatment, the EECP device was operated at a pressure of 0.019–0.029 MPa, with each session lasting 45 minutes, performed 3 to 5 times per week. Hemodynamic parameters were measured at three time points: before EECP, after 17 hours of EECP, and following the final 35-hour EECP session, using color Doppler ultrasound [38].

The results showed that after 35 hours of EECP, EDV in the left and right CCA significantly increased; RI significantly decreased; The FR in the left CCA also considerably increased (767.659 ± 105.02 vs. 692.798 ± 125.925 cm/s, $p = 0.021$). In addition, the frequency-domain features of the CCA—second peak (y_2) and power spectral energy ratio at 2.05 Hz (PSER (2.05 Hz)) showed significant differences after 35 h-EECP, as well as between 17 h and 35 h-EECP sessions. Following both 17-hour and 35-hour EECP interventions, the brachial artery FR increased significantly. After 35 h of EECP, the ID and FR of the femoral artery also showed significant improvement. Moreover, after 17 h of EECP, the PSER (2.05 Hz) in the right CCA increased significantly, although peak frequency and very-low-frequency spectral energy ratios did not show statistically significant changes [38].

These findings suggest that changes in EDV, ID, RI, and FR of the CCA reflect hemodynamic alterations in the neck region, which may serve as early indicators for cervical vascular disease and coronary artery disease [98]. In this study, long-term EECP treatment significantly enhanced EDV, ID, and FR, suggesting improved vascular elasticity, enhanced diastolic function, and increased blood flow and perfusion [99, 100]. Additionally, EECP reduced vascular resistance in the distal carotid artery, particularly in cerebral circulation, thereby improving cerebral perfusion [101]. Changes in peripheral vessel diameter and diastolic function further supported increased peripheral perfusion [99]. Moreover, changes in frequency-domain characteristics provided important evidence of the long-term effects of EECP. In particular, the y_2 and PSER (2.05 Hz) parameters of the CCA exhibited notable alterations. Frequency-domain indices have been shown to reflect not only arterial hemodynamic changes but also disease-related information such as arteriosclerosis and increased peripheral resistance [95, 102]. Specifically, y_2, as a peak-related descriptor, reflects blood flow waveform changes during diastole. Previous studies have indicated that low-frequency components in the spectral domain carry rich information about waveform variability. Thus, the observed changes in PSER (2.05 Hz) in this study further support the theoretical foundation for using frequency-domain features in disease analysis and hemodynamic assessment.

5.3 The predictive value of hemodynamic features

The transfer function of a system plays a significant predictive role in evaluating hemodynamic changes. In mathematical modeling of the cardiovascular system, this method treats the entire circulatory system as a nonlinear black box and uses system identification techniques—such as maximum likelihood estimation or the least squares method—to estimate the relationship between system inputs and outputs, thereby revealing the system's physiological characteristics. This approach has been widely applied in the analysis of physiological signals such as electrocardiography (ECG), electroencephalography (EEG), and electromyography (EMG). Research shows that the transfer function not only reflects cerebral autoregulation but also captures changes in vascular properties. Thus, this section aims to explore whether the transfer function between arteries under EECP stimulation can reflect differences between CAD patients and healthy controls, thereby providing a theoretical basis for dynamic mechanism exploration and disease assessment from a novel perspective [103].

Based on quality-controlled spectral data, transfer functions were computed for 50 CAD patients and 50 healthy controls, using ultrasound blood flow velocity spectra recorded from the CCA to the brachial artery, at three EECP stages: before, during, and after intervention.

Model order was selected using final prediction error (FPE) criteria, and a 12th-order autoregressive with exogenous input (ARX) model was adopted. From each transfer function, 73 features were extracted, including: Model coefficients (A and B), Real and imaginary parts of zeros and poles. Across three EECP states, this yielded a total of 219 transfer function features per subject [103].

To reduce dimensionality and identify discriminative features, three feature selection algorithms were applied: Stepwise regression, Correlation-based Feature Selection (CFS), and Lasso regression. Each method identified key features that

Feature selection algorithm	Coefficients selected	Zeros selected	Poles selected	Classification accuracy (SVM + 10-Fold CV)
Stepwise Regression	1	3	66%	66%
CFS	2	4	68%	68%
Lasso Regression	1	5	73%	73%

Table 1.
Feature selection results and classification accuracy.

distinguished between the two groups. The ability of these features to classify CAD vs. control groups was evaluated using support vector machine (SVM) classifiers with 10-fold cross-validation (**Table 1**) [103].

Results indicate that using the 12th-order ARX transfer function model, hemodynamic transfer characteristics from the CCA to the brachial artery can effectively differentiate between CAD patients and healthy controls. Among the three algorithms, Lasso regression achieved the highest accuracy (73%), suggesting its strong potential for predictive modeling in cardiovascular rehabilitation. Notably, zeros and poles were repeatedly selected across algorithms, underscoring their role in capturing functional hemodynamic differences between the two groups. Overall, these features demonstrated high sensitivity to dynamic changes, and their consistent selection and classification performance support their clinical utility in disease prediction and rehabilitation assessment [103].

5.4 Hemodynamic analysis based on 0D-1D model

Hemodynamic simulation offers unique potential and advantages in uncovering the underlying mechanisms of the therapeutic effects induced by EECP. Although several studies have attempted to investigate the hemodynamic effects of EECP using computational fluid dynamics (CFD) or fluid–structure interaction models, these studies often suffer from limitations, such as oversimplified model structures that fail to capture the global rheological changes induced by EECP, or reliance on partial clinical data from only a few vascular segments. At present, there is a lack of comprehensive predictive approaches specifically targeting the hemodynamic improvements associated with EECP. This includes a shortage of individualized simulation methods, and more critically, an absence of systematic integration of CFD simulation and clinical validation to explore the relationship between optimal EECP protocols and patient-specific vascular parameters. This section aims to bridge this gap by employing hemodynamic simulation to explain the mechanisms behind phenomena observed during clinical EECP interventions. The final objective is to validate the simulation findings using clinical measurements, ensuring the practical relevance of the study [104].

A siphon model (SM) was developed using ultrasound imaging data, focusing on resting and EECP states. Parameters such as femoral artery blood flow and PWV were analyzed to reveal how cuff pressure modulates femoral flow dynamics. In parallel, a patient-specific 0D–1D model was constructed using personalized ultrasound-based anatomical and flow parameters from the aorta (AO), femoral artery (FA), and brachial artery (BA) at rest. This model was then coupled with the siphon model to simulate hemodynamic responses under various EECP conditions. Finally, simulation outputs were compared against clinical measurements during EECP to assess model

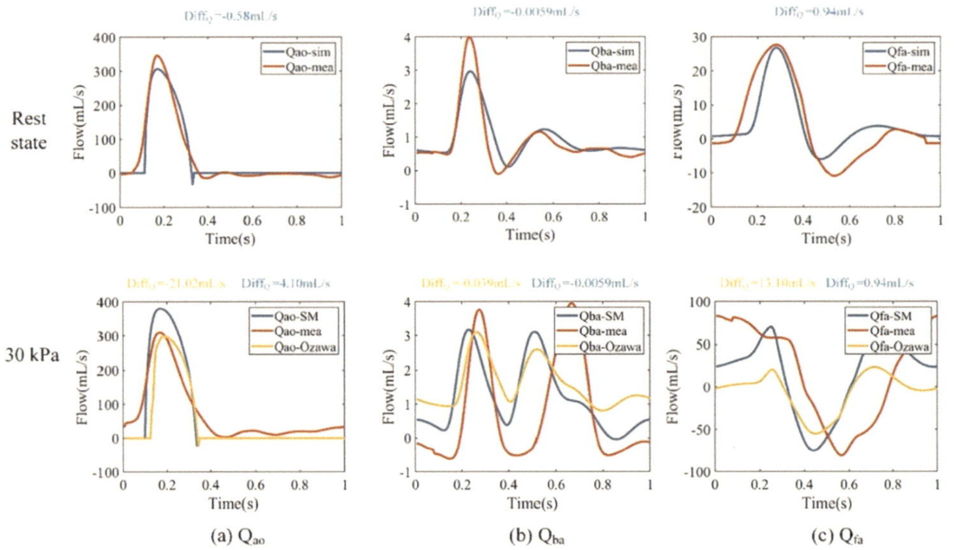

Figure 10.
The clinical measurements were compared with the outputs of the personalized model in the rest state (upper), and the personalized model, coupled with our proposed model and Ozawa's model, was compared with clinical measurements in the EECP state (lower) [82]. (Source: https://www.sciencedirect.com/science/article/pii/S0021929024001349?via%3Dihub&__cf_chl_tk=iTC8YZpc_NfRgwYcZoZKZmrjC8gR4MVJx9dVzJuBWLs-1773749124-1.0.1.1-8emY4YaEOZxRnj4PANlpHkvsoSgt6Xrk8gxlUbjoF_E).

accuracy and validate the underlying hypotheses [82]. The overall research workflow is illustrated in **Figure 9**.

A clinical trial was conducted involving 24 volunteers—15 healthy subjects and 9 patients with CAD. Each participant underwent EECP treatment at four different cuff pressure levels: 20, 25, 30, and 35 kPa. Lower limb vascular blood flow data were collected at rest and under each pressure condition. The simulated outputs of the coupled 0D–1D model were compared with actual clinical measurements taken during EECP sessions to validate the model's accuracy in predicting real-time hemodynamic responses. To further demonstrate the superiority of the proposed model in predicting blood flow dynamics, the measured flow waveforms were compared with the predicted results from Ozawa's model and the predictions from our personalized coupled model. The comparative results are shown in **Figure 10** [82].

Clinical findings demonstrated that during diastole, there was a substantial centripetal (retrograde) blood flow in the femoral artery (FA), while during systole, significant forward flow was observed from the aorta (AO) to the peripheral arteries. Notably, these hemodynamic changes were not captured by Ozawa's model, whereas the siphon model (SM) effectively described these variations throughout the entire cardiac cycle (see **Figure 10(c)**) [82]. This highlights the clinical relevance and accuracy of the proposed model and coupling strategy in representing FA hemodynamics.

6. Conclusion(s)

This chapter consists of five parts. The first part includes the definitions of cardiac rehabilitation and health promotion, as well as the methods and approaches of exercise rehabilitation. The second part presents the principles of methods, including hemodynamics, blood flow, and pulse wave. The third, fourth, and fifth parts respectively relied on hemodynamic analysis and multimodal physiological indicators to study the effects of different exercise modes on cardiovascular disease, the response of passive exercise-EECP to cardiovascular function, and to identify the optimal blood flow indicators for personalized treatment.

In this chapter, we firstly found that CPET revealed clear hemodynamic differences between UHS and HS: SDPPG response: Post-CPET, b/a, and AGI were significantly higher in UHS, while d/a and c/a were lower, suggesting exercise stress unveils subclinical arterial stiffness and microvascular dysfunction in UHS. PPG morphology and multiparametric interaction: During CPET, UHS exhibited greater BP elevation, abnormal LF/HF heart rate variability, and PTT changes, indicating impaired cardiovascular compensation. CPET provides objective metrics for early risk stratification.

Secondly, meta-analysis of 38 studies involving 2089 CVD patients showed that aerobic training significantly reduces central systolic pressure, cf-PWV, and improves cardiac output and LVEF. Resistance training effectively lowers ASP and central diastolic pressure. Combined training improves cf-PWV and CO but may increase AIx. Among all modes, aerobic training demonstrates the strongest evidence in improving arterial stiffness and cardiac function, while resistance training uniquely benefits central blood pressure regulation.

Thirdly, we found that a single session of EECP expands brachial/femoral artery diameters, reduces carotid RI, and alters frequency-domain features, indicating blood flow redistribution. Moreover, after long-term EECP, significant increases in carotid EDV and flow rate (FR) were observed, indicating improved vascular elasticity and perfusion. Furthermore, transfer function features (pole-zero coordinates) used in an SVM classifier distinguished CAD from healthy subjects with up to 73% accuracy. 0D–1D coupled modeling: Patient-specific simulations accurately predicted femoral artery hemodynamic responses under EECP, providing a robust theoretical basis for personalized treatment planning.

In summary, through multi-modal hemodynamic evaluation, this study systematically demonstrated the mechanistic improvements in cardiovascular function through both active (exercise-based) and passive (EECP) rehabilitation strategies. Aerobic training remains the most effective core intervention for central hemodynamics optimization and arterial stiffness reversal. Meanwhile, EECP, as a passive modality, promotes vascular repair via hemodynamic redistribution. By integrating computational modeling and non-invasive monitoring, this research provides a scientific and practical foundation for the precision implementation of cardiovascular rehabilitation.

Acknowledgements

This work was, in part, supported by the National Natural Science Foundation of China [Grant No. 82202292], National Key Research and Development Program of China (NO.2025YFF0518400). Part of this research was supported by Guangdong Medical Science and Technology Research Foundation (No. A2022383) and Guangdong Basic and Applied Research Foundation (No.2021A1515110738).

Conflict of interest

The Authors declare that there is no conflict of interest.

Author details

Yahui Zhang[1]*, Xiaodong Zhang[2], Chaoyang Wang[3] and Kai Liu[4]

1 School of Rehabilitation Sciences and Engineering, University of Health and Rehabilitation Sciences, Shandong Province, China

2 Department of Public Education, University of Health and Rehabilitation Sciences, Shandong Province, China

3 Graduate School, Harbin Sport University, Harbin, China

4 Department of Cardiology, Qingdao Hospital, University of Health and Rehabilitation Sciences (Qingdao Municipal Hospital), Qingdao, China

*Address all correspondence to: zyh1171518067@163.com

References

[1] Piepoli MF, Corrà U, Benzer W, Bjarnason-Wehrens B, Dendale P, Gaita D, et al. Secondary prevention through cardiac rehabilitation: From knowledge to implementation. A position paper from the cardiac rehabilitation section of the European Association of Cardiovascular Prevention and Rehabilitation. European Journal of Cardiovascular Prevention and Rehabilitation. 2010;**17**(1):11-17

[2] Thomas RJ, King M, Lui K, Oldridge N, Piña IL, Spertus J, et al. AACVPR/ACC/AHA 2007 performance measures on cardiac rehabilitation for referral to and delivery of cardiac rehabilitation/secondary prevention services endorsed by the American College of Chest Physicians, American College of Sports Medicine, American Physical Therapy Association, Canadian Association of Cardiac Rehabilitation, European Association for Cardiovascular Prevention and Rehabilitation, inter-American Heart Foundation, National Association of clinical nurse specialists, preventive cardiovascular nurses association, and the Society of Thoracic Surgeons. Journal of the American College of Cardiology. 2007;**50**(14): 1400-1433

[3] Koller A, Laughlin MH, Cenko E, de Wit C, Tóth K, Bugiardini R, et al. Functional and structural adaptations of the coronary macro- and microvasculature to regular aerobic exercise by activation of physiological, cellular, and molecular mechanisms: ESC working group on coronary pathophysiology and microcirculation position paper. Cardiovascular Research. 2022;**118**(2):357-371

[4] Lixia Yuan RD. Interpretation of the guidelines for cardiac rehabilitation and secondary prevention in China. Chinese Circulation Journal. 2019;**34** (S1):86-90

[5] Long L, Mordi IR, Bridges C, Sagar VA, Davies EJ, Coats AJ, et al. Exercise-based cardiac rehabilitation for adults with heart failure. Cochrane Database of Systematic Reviews. 2019; **1**(1):Cd003331

[6] Wang H, Li Y, Chai K, Long Z, Yang Z, Du M, et al. Mortality in patients admitted to hospital with heart failure in China: A nationwide cardiovascular association database-heart failure Centre registry cohort study. The Lancet Global Health. 2024;**12**(4):e611-e622

[7] Organization WH. Ottawa Charter for Health Promotion. Geneva, Switzerland: WHO; 1986

[8] Puska P, Jaini P. The North Karelia project: Prevention of cardiovascular disease in Finland through population-based lifestyle interventions. American Journal of Lifestyle Medicine. 2020; **14**(5):495-499

[9] WHO Expert Committee on Rehabilitation after Cardiovascular Diseases, with Special Emphasis on Developing Countries. Rehabilitation after cardiovascular diseases, with special emphasis on developing countries. Report of a WHO expert committee. World Health Organization Technical Report Series. 1993;**831**:1-122

[10] Balady GJ, Williams MA, Ades PA, Bittner V, Comoss P, Foody JM, et al. Core components of cardiac rehabilitation/secondary prevention programs: 2007 update: A scientific statement from the American Heart Association exercise, cardiac rehabilitation, and prevention committee, the council on clinical

cardiology; the councils on cardiovascular nursing, epidemiology and prevention, and nutrition, physical activity, and metabolism; and the American Association of Cardiovascular and Pulmonary Rehabilitation. Circulation. 2007;**115**(20):2675-2682

[11] Fihn SD, Blankenship JC, Alexander KP, Bittl JA, Byrne JG, Fletcher BJ, et al. 2014 ACC/AHA/AATS/PCNA/SCAI/STS focused update of the guideline for the diagnosis and management of patients with stable ischemic heart disease: A report of the American College of Cardiology/American Heart Association task force on practice guidelines, and the American Association for Thoracic Surgery, preventive cardiovascular nurses association, Society for Cardiovascular Angiography and Interventions, and Society of Thoracic Surgeons. Journal of the American College of Cardiology. 2014;**64**(18):1929-1949

[12] Mezzani A, Hamm LF, Jones AM, McBride PE, Moholdt T, Stone JA, et al. Aerobic exercise intensity assessment and prescription in cardiac rehabilitation: A joint position statement of the European Association for Cardiovascular Prevention and Rehabilitation, the American Association of Cardiovascular and Pulmonary Rehabilitation, and the Canadian Association of Cardiac Rehabilitation. Journal of Cardiopulmonary Rehabilitation and Prevention. 2012; **32**(6):327-350

[13] Zheng ZS, Li TM, Kambic H, Chen GH, Yu LQ, Cai SR, et al. Sequential external counterpulsation (SECP) in China. Transactions - American Society for Artificial Internal Organs. 1983;**29**:599-603

[14] Lawson WE, Hui JC, Soroff HS, Zheng ZS, Kayden DS, Sasvary D, et al. Efficacy of enhanced external counterpulsation in the treatment of angina pectoris. The American Journal of Cardiology. 1992;**70**(9):859-862

[15] Montalescot G, Sechtem U, Achenbach S, Andreotti F, Arden C, Budaj A, et al. 2013 ESC guidelines on the management of stable coronary artery disease: The task force on the management of stable coronary artery disease of the European Society of Cardiology. European Heart Journal. 2013;**34**(38):2949-3003

[16] Mielniczuk L, da Silva LB, Haddad H. Enhanced external counterpulsation in ischemic heart disease and congestive heart failure. CMAJ. 2004;**170**(8):1223-1224

[17] Yin Q, Jiang H, Zhang Z, Zhang L, Wu Z, Huang L, et al. Influence of enhanced external counterpulsation on endothelial function: A meta-analysis of randomized controlled trials. Scandinavian Cardiovascular Journal. 2023;**57**(1):2273223

[18] Secomb TW. Hemodynamics. Comprehensive Physiology. 2016;**6**(2): 975-1003

[19] Liu D. Thirty years of clinical hemodynamics. Medical Journal of Peking Union Medical College Hospital. 2019;**10**(5):433-437

[20] Allen J. Photoplethysmography and its application in clinical physiological measurement. Physiological Measurement. 2007;**28**(3):R1-R39

[21] Shah A, Irshad A. Sonography doppler flow imaging instrumentation. In: StatPearls. Treasure Island (FL): StatPearls Publishing, LLC; 2025

[22] Soleimani E, Mokhtari-Dizaji M, Fatouraee N, Saberi H. Assessing the blood pressure waveform of the carotid

artery using an ultrasound image processing method. Ultrasonography. 2017;**36**(2):144-152

[23] Tang J, Kilic K, Szabo TL, Boas DA. Improved color Doppler for cerebral blood flow axial velocity imaging. IEEE Transactions on Medical Imaging. 2021; **40**(2):758-764

[24] Townsend RR, Wilkinson IB, Schiffrin EL, Avolio AP, Chirinos JA, Cockcroft JR, et al. Recommendations for improving and standardizing vascular research on arterial stiffness: A scientific statement from the American Heart Association. Hypertension. 2015; **66**(3):698-722

[25] Min S, An J, Lee JH, Kim JH, Joe DJ, Eom SH, et al. Wearable blood pressure sensors for cardiovascular monitoring and machine learning algorithms for blood pressure estimation. Nature Reviews. Cardiology. 2025;**22**(9): 629-648

[26] Kim HL. Arterial stiffness and hypertension. Clinical Hypertension. 2023;**29**(1):31

[27] Pilz N, Heinz V, Ax T, Fesseler L, Patzak A, Bothe TL. Pulse wave velocity: Methodology, clinical applications, and interplay with heart rate variability. Reviews in Cardiovascular Medicine. 2024;**25**(7):266

[28] Chang YW, Hsiu H, Yang SH, Fang WH, Tsai HC. Characteristics of beat-to-beat photoplethysmography waveform indexes in subjects with metabolic syndrome. Microvascular Research. 2016;**106**:80-87

[29] Minhas A, Pal SC, Jain K. Machine learning analysis of integrated ABP and PPG signals towards early detection of coronary artery disease. Scientific Reports. 2025;**15**(1):8574

[30] Weng WH, Baur S, Daswani M, Chen C, Harrell L, Kakarmath S, et al. Predicting cardiovascular disease risk using photoplethysmography and deep learning. PLOS Global Public Health. 2024;**4**(6):e0003204

[31] Dall'Olio L, Curti N, Remondini D, Safi Harb Y, Asselbergs FW, Castellani G, et al. Prediction of vascular aging based on smartphone acquired PPG signals. Scientific Reports. 2020; **10**(1):19756

[32] Hashimoto J, Chonan K, Aoki Y, Nishimura T, Ohkubo T, Hozawa A, et al. Pulse wave velocity and the second derivative of the finger photoplethysmogram in treated hypertensive patients: Their relationship and associating factors. Journal of Hypertension. 2002;**20**(12): 2415-2422

[33] Elgendi M. On the analysis of fingertip photoplethysmogram signals. Current Cardiology Reviews. 2012;**8**(1): 14-25

[34] Takazawa K, Tanaka N, Fujita M, Matsuoka O, Saiki T, Aikawa M, et al. Assessment of vasoactive agents and vascular aging by the second derivative of photoplethysmogram waveform. Hypertension. 1998;**32**(2): 365-370

[35] Laukkanen JA, Rauramaa R. Systolic blood pressure during exercise testing and the risk of sudden cardiac death. International Journal of Cardiology. 2013;**168**(3):3046-3047

[36] Otsuka T, Kawada T, Katsumata M, Ibuki C, Kusama Y. Independent determinants of second derivative of the finger photoplethysmogram among various cardiovascular risk factors in middle-aged men. Hypertension Research. 2007;**30**(12):1211-1218

[37] Yousef Q, Reaz MBI, Ali MAM. The analysis of PPG morphology: Investigating the effects of aging on arterial compliance. Measurement Science Review. 2012;**12**(6):266

[38] Zhang Y. Research on Key Issues of Exercise-Based Cardiac Rehabilitation Based on Multiple Physiological Signal Analysis. Shenyang, Liaoning Province, China: Northeastern University; 2020

[39] Zhang Y, Jiang Z, Qi L, Xu L, Sun X, Chu X, et al. Evaluation of cardiorespiratory function during cardiopulmonary exercise testing in untreated hypertensive and healthy subjects. Frontiers in Physiology. 2018;**9**: 1590. DOI: 10.3389/fphys.2018.01590/full

[40] Imanaga I, Hara H, Koyanagi S, Tanaka K. Correlation between wave components of the second derivative of plethysmogram and arterial distensibility. Japanese Heart Journal. 1998;**39**(6):775-784

[41] Hafifah A, Anuar NN. Methods of extracting feature from photoplethysmogram waveform for non-invasive diagnostic applications. International Journal of Online and Biomedical Engineering. 2020;**16**: 39-62

[42] Ovadia-Blechman Z, Hauptman Y, Rabin N, Wiezman G, Hoffer O, Gertz SD, et al. Morphological features of the photoplethysmographic signal: A new approach to characterize the microcirculatory response to photobiomodulation. Frontiers in Physiology. 2023;**14**:1175470

[43] Dominguez-Rodriguez A, Arroyo-Ucar E, Abreu-Gonzalez P, Tome MC, Hernandez-Garcia C, Del Carmen G-BM, et al. Cardiopulmonary exercise testing and prognostic assessment of hypertensive cardiomyopathy: An emerging application. International Journal of Cardiology. 2013; **167**(5):2368-2370

[44] Nikolic SB, Sharman JE, Adams MJ, Edwards LM. Metabolomics in hypertension. Journal of Hypertension. 2014;**32**(6):1159-1169

[45] Cockcroft JR, Webb DJ, Wilkinson IB. Arterial stiffness, hypertension and diabetes mellitus. Journal of Human Hypertension. 2000; **14**(6):377-380

[46] Wibmer T, Doering K, Kropf-Sanchen C, Rüdiger S, Blanta I, Stoiber KM, et al. Pulse transit time and blood pressure during cardiopulmonary exercise tests. Physiological Research. 2014;**63**(3):287-296

[47] Rivas-Vilchis JF, Hernández-Sánchez F, González-Camarena R, Suárez-Rodríguez LD, Escorcia-Gaona R, Cervantes-Reyes JA, et al. Assessment of the vascular effects of PC6 (Neiguan) using the second derivative of the finger photoplethysmogram in healthy and hypertensive subjects. The American Journal of Chinese Medicine. 2007;**35**(3): 427-436

[48] Tabara Y, Igase M, Okada Y, Nagai T, Miki T, Ohyagi Y, et al. Usefulness of the second derivative of the finger photoplethysmogram for assessment of end-organ damage: The J-SHIPP study. Hypertension Research. 2016;**39**(7):552-556

[49] Kohjitani A, Miyata M, Iwase Y, Ohno S, Tohya A, Manabe Y, et al. Associations between the autonomic nervous system and the second derivative of the finger photoplethysmogram indices. Journal of Atherosclerosis and Thrombosis. 2014;**21**(5):501-508

[50] Mohamad Rozi R, Usman S, Mohd Ali MA, Reaz MBI. Second derivatives of

photoplethysmography (PPG) for estimating vascular aging of atherosclerotic patients. In: 2012 IEEE-EMBS Conference on Biomedical Engineering and Sciences. Langkawi, Malaysia: IEEE; 2012. pp. 256-259

[51] Mensah GA, Fuster V, Murray CJL, Roth GA. Global burden of cardiovascular diseases and risks, 1990-2022. Journal of the American College of Cardiology. 2023; **82**(25):2350-2473

[52] Feigin VL, Brainin M, Norrving B, Martins SO, Pandian J, Lindsay P, et al. World stroke organization: Global stroke fact sheet 2025. International Journal of Stroke. 2025;**20**(2):132-144

[53] Mendis S, Davis S, Norrving B. Organizational update: The world health organization global status report on noncommunicable diseases 2014; one more landmark step in the combat against stroke and vascular disease. Stroke. 2015;**46**(5): e121-e122

[54] Kohl HW 3rd, Craig CL, Lambert EV, Inoue S, Alkandari JR, Leetongin G, et al. The pandemic of physical inactivity: Global action for public health. Lancet. 2012;**380**(9838): 294-305

[55] Dans A, Ng N, Varghese C, Tai ES, Firestone R, Bonita R. The rise of chronic non-communicable diseases in Southeast Asia: Time for action. Lancet. 2011; **377**(9766):680-689

[56] Vanhees L, Rauch B, Piepoli M, van Buuren F, Takken T, Börjesson M, et al. Importance of characteristics and modalities of physical activity and exercise in the management of cardiovascular health in individuals with cardiovascular disease (Part III). European Journal of Preventive Cardiology. 2012;**19**(6):1333-1356

[57] Zhang Y, Qi L, Xu L, Sun X, Liu W, Zhou S, et al. Effects of exercise modalities on central hemodynamics, arterial stiffness and cardiac function in cardiovascular disease: Systematic review and meta-analysis of randomized controlled trials. PLoS One. 2018;**13**(7): e0200829. DOI: 10.1371/journal.pone.0200829

[58] Nichols WW, Orourke MF, Vlachopoulos C. Mcdonald's Blood Flow in Arteries: Theoretical, Experimental and Clinical Principles. 6th ed. London: Arnold; 2011

[59] Roman MJ, Devereux RB, Kizer JR, Lee ET, Galloway JM, Ali T, et al. Central pressure more strongly relates to vascular disease and outcome than does brachial pressure: The Strong Heart Study. Hypertension. 2007;**50**(1):197-203

[60] Wang KL, Cheng HM, Chuang SY, Spurgeon HA, Ting CT, Lakatta EG, et al. Central or peripheral systolic or pulse pressure: Which best relates to target organs and future mortality? Journal of Hypertension. 2009;**27**(3):461-467

[61] Davies JE, Baksi J, Francis DP, Hadjiloizou N, Whinnett ZI, Manisty CH, et al. The arterial reservoir pressure increases with aging and is the major determinant of the aortic augmentation index. American Journal of Physiology. Heart and Circulatory Physiology. 2010;**298**(2):H580-H586

[62] Laurent S, Cockcroft J, Van Bortel L, Boutouyrie P, Giannattasio C, Hayoz D, et al. Expert consensus document on arterial stiffness: Methodological issues and clinical applications. European Heart Journal. 2006;**27**(21):2588-2605

[63] Heffernan KS, Yoon ES, Sharman JE, Davies JE, Shih YT, Chen CH, et al. Resistance exercise training reduces arterial reservoir pressure in older adults

with prehypertension and hypertension. Hypertension Research. 2013;**36**(5): 422-427

[64] Ashor AW, Lara J, Siervo M, Celis-Morales C, Mathers JC. Effects of exercise modalities on arterial stiffness and wave reflection: A systematic review and meta-analysis of randomized controlled trials. PLoS One. 2014;**9**(10): e110034

[65] Stöhr EJ, McDonnell B, Thompson J, Stone K, Bull T, Houston R, et al. Left ventricular mechanics in humans with high aerobic fitness: Adaptation independent of structural remodelling, arterial haemodynamics and heart rate. The Journal of Physiology. 2012;**590**(9): 2107-2119

[66] Mitchell GF, Conlin PR, Dunlap ME, Lacourcière Y, Arnold JM, Ogilvie RI, et al. Aortic diameter, wall stiffness, and wave reflection in systolic hypertension. Hypertension. 2008;**51**(1):105-111

[67] Montero D, Vinet A, Roberts CK. Effect of combined aerobic and resistance training versus aerobic training on arterial stiffness. International Journal of Cardiology. 2015;**178**:69-76

[68] Huang C, Wang J, Deng S, She Q, Wu L. The effects of aerobic endurance exercise on pulse wave velocity and intima media thickness in adults: A systematic review and meta-analysis. Scandinavian Journal of Medicine & Science in Sports. 2016;**26**(5): 478-487

[69] Donley DA, Fournier SB, Reger BL, DeVallance E, Bonner DE, Olfert IM, et al. Aerobic exercise training reduces arterial stiffness in metabolic syndrome. Journal of Applied Physiology (Bethesda, MD: 1985). 2014;**116**(11):1396-1404

[70] Gladden JD, Linke WA, Redfield MM. Heart failure with preserved ejection fraction. Pflügers Archiv. 2014;**466**(6):1037-1053

[71] Haykowsky MJ, Liang Y, Pechter D, Jones LW, McAlister FA, Clark AM. A meta-analysis of the effect of exercise training on left ventricular remodeling in heart failure patients: The benefit depends on the type of training performed. Journal of the American College of Cardiology. 2007;**49**(24):2329-2336

[72] Cheetham C, Green D, Collis J, Dembo L, O'Driscoll G. Effect of aerobic and resistance exercise on central hemodynamic responses in severe chronic heart failure. Journal of Applied Physiology (Bethesda, MD: 1985). 2002; **93**(1):175-180

[73] Coats AJ, Adamopoulos S, Radaelli A, McCance A, Meyer TE, Bernardi L, et al. Controlled trial of physical training in chronic heart failure. Exercise performance, hemodynamics, ventilation, and autonomic function. Circulation. 1992;**85**(6):2119-2131

[74] Belardinelli R, Georgiou D, Ginzton L, Cianci G, Purcaro A. Effects of moderate exercise training on thallium uptake and contractile response to low-dose dobutamine of dysfunctional myocardium in patients with ischemic cardiomyopathy. Circulation. 1998; **97**(6):553-561

[75] Miyachi M, Kawano H, Sugawara J, Takahashi K, Hayashi K, Yamazaki K, et al. Unfavorable effects of resistance training on central arterial compliance: A randomized intervention study. Circulation. 2004;**110**(18):2858-2863

[76] Kawano H, Tanimoto M, Yamamoto K, Sanada K, Gando Y, Tabata I, et al. Resistance training in men is associated with increased arterial

stiffness and blood pressure but does not adversely affect endothelial function as measured by arterial reactivity to the cold pressor test. Experimental Physiology. 2008;**93**(2):296-302

[77] Wildman RP, Mackey RH, Bostom A, Thompson T, Sutton-Tyrrell K. Measures of obesity are associated with vascular stiffness in young and older adults. Hypertension. 2003;**42**(4): 468-473

[78] Croymans DM, Krell SL, Oh CS, Katiraie M, Lam CY, Harris RA, et al. Effects of resistance training on central blood pressure in obese young men. Journal of Human Hypertension. 2014; **28**(3):157-164

[79] Figueroa A. Effects of resistance training on central blood pressure and wave reflection in obese adults with prehypertension. Journal of Human Hypertension. 2014;**28**(3):143-144

[80] Taaffe DR, Galvão DA, Sharman JE, Coombes JS. Reduced central blood pressure in older adults following progressive resistance training. Journal of Human Hypertension. 2007;**21**(1): 96-98

[81] Parker KH, Alastruey J, Stan GB. Arterial reservoir-excess pressure and ventricular work. Medical & Biological Engineering & Computing. 2012;**50**(4): 419-424

[82] Zhang Q, Zhang YH, Hao LL, Xu XH, Wu GF, Lin L, et al. A numerical study on the siphonic effect of enhanced external counterpulsation at lower extremities with a coupled 0D-1D closed-loop personalized hemodynamics model. Journal of Biomechanics. 2024;**166**:112057. Available from: https://www.sciencedirect.com/science/article/pii/S0021929024001349?via%3Dihub&__cf_chl_tk=iTC8YZpc_NfRgwYcZoZKZmrjC8gR4MVJx9dVzJuBWLs-1773749124-1.0.1.1-8emY4YaEOZxRnj4PANlpHkvsoSgt6Xrk8gxlUbj0F_E

[83] Fu TC, Wang CH, Lin PS, Hsu CC, Cherng WJ, Huang SC, et al. Aerobic interval training improves oxygen uptake efficiency by enhancing cerebral and muscular hemodynamics in patients with heart failure. International Journal of Cardiology. 2013;**167**(1):41-50

[84] Van Craenenbroeck AH, Van Craenenbroeck EM, Van Ackeren K, Vrints CJ, Conraads VM, Verpooten GA, et al. Effect of moderate aerobic exercise training on endothelial function and arterial stiffness in CKD stages 3-4: A randomized controlled trial. American Journal of Kidney Diseases. 2015;**66**(2): 285-296

[85] Crisafulli A, Piras F, Filippi M, Piredda C, Chiappori P, Melis F, et al. Role of heart rate and stroke volume during muscle metaboreflex-induced cardiac output increase: Differences between activation during and after exercise. The Journal of Physiological Sciences. 2011;**61**(5):385-394

[86] Miyachi M. Effects of resistance training on arterial stiffness: A meta-analysis. British Journal of Sports Medicine. 2013;**47**(6):393-396

[87] Li Y, Hanssen H, Cordes M, Rossmeissl A, Endes S, Schmidt-Trucksäss A. Aerobic, resistance and combined exercise training on arterial stiffness in normotensive and hypertensive adults: A review. European Journal of Sport Science. 2015;**15**(5): 443-457

[88] Brown MD, Dengel DR, Hogikyan RV, Supiano MA. Sympathetic activity and the heterogenous blood pressure response to exercise training in hypertensives. Journal of Applied

Physiology (Bethesda, MD: 1985). 2002; **92**(4):1434-1442

[89] Lee YH, Park SH, Yoon ES, Lee CD, Wee SO, Fernhall B, et al. Effects of combined aerobic and resistance exercise on central arterial stiffness and gait velocity in patients with chronic poststroke hemiparesis. American Journal of Physical Medicine & Rehabilitation. 2015;**94**(9):687-695

[90] Beck DT, Martin JS, Casey DP, Braith RW. Exercise training reduces peripheral arterial stiffness and myocardial oxygen demand in young prehypertensive subjects. American Journal of Hypertension. 2013;**26**(9): 1093-1102

[91] Oliveira NL, Ribeiro F, Silva G, Alves AJ, Silva N, Guimarães JT, et al. Effect of exercise-based cardiac rehabilitation on arterial stiffness and inflammatory and endothelial dysfunction biomarkers: A randomized controlled trial of myocardial infarction patients. Atherosclerosis. 2015;**239**(1): 150-157

[92] Ozawa ET, Bottom KE, Xiao X, Kamm RD. Numerical simulation of enhanced external counterpulsation. Annals of Biomedical Engineering. 2001; **29**(4):284-297

[93] Zhang Y, Chen Z, Mai Z, Zhou W, Wang H, Zhang X, et al. Acute hemodynamic responses to enhanced external counterpulsation in patients with coronary artery disease. Frontiers in Cardiovascular Medicine. 2021;**8**:721140

[94] Krause H, Segard M, Carey P, Bernstein EF, Fronek A. Doppler power frequency spectrum analysis in the diagnosis of carotid artery disease. Stroke. 1984;**15**(2):351-358

[95] Agnew CE, McCann AJ, Lockhart CJ, Hamilton PK, McVeigh GE, McGivern RC. Comparison of rootMUSIC and discrete wavelet transform analysis of Doppler ultrasound blood flow waveforms to detect microvascular abnormalities in type I diabetes. IEEE Transactions on Biomedical Engineering. 2011;**58**(4): 861-867

[96] Ferreira LF, Harper AJ, Barstow TJ. Frequency-domain characteristics and filtering of blood flow following the onset of exercise: Implications for kinetics analysis. Journal of Applied Physiology (Bethesda, MD: 1985). 2006; **100**(3):817-825

[97] Perini R, Orizio C, Baselli G, Cerutti S, Veicsteinas A. The influence of exercise intensity on the power spectrum of heart rate variability. European Journal of Applied Physiology and Occupational Physiology. 1990;**61**(1–2): 143-148

[98] Bai CH, Chen JR, Chiu HC, Pan WH. Lower blood flow velocity, higher resistance index, and larger diameter of extracranial carotid arteries are associated with ischemic stroke independently of carotid atherosclerosis and cardiovascular risk factors. Journal of Clinical Ultrasound. 2007;**35**(6): 322-330

[99] Järhult SJ, Sundström J, Lind L. Brachial artery hyperemic blood flow velocities are related to carotid atherosclerosis. Clinical Physiology and Functional Imaging. 2009;**29**(5):360-365

[100] Kallikazaros I, Tsioufis C, Sideris S, Stefanadis C, Toutouzas P. Carotid artery disease as a marker for the presence of severe coronary artery disease in patients evaluated for chest pain. Stroke. 1999;**30**(5):1002-1007

[101] Frauchiger B, Schmid HP, Roedel C, Moosmann P, Staub D. Comparison of

carotid arterial resistive indices with intima-media thickness as sonographic markers of atherosclerosis. Stroke. 2001; **32**(4):836-841

[102] Avolio A, Westerhof BE, Siebes M, Tyberg JV. Arterial hemodynamics and wave analysis in the frequency and time domains: An evaluation of the paradigms. Medical & Biological Engineering & Computing. 2009;**47**(2): 107-110

[103] Zhang Y, Yang D, Zhao X, Luo Y, Wang Y, Zhong C. Vascular ultrasound data during enhanced external counterpulsation for predicting coronary artery disease. Annual International Conference of the IEEE Engineering in Medicine and Biology Society. 2025; **2025**:1-5

[104] Zhang Q, Zhang Y, Hao L, Zhong Y, Wu K, Wang Z, et al. A personalized 0D-1D model of cardiovascular system for the hemodynamic simulation of enhanced external counterpulsation. Computer Methods and Programs in Biomedicine. 2022;**227**:107224

Section 2

Exercise for Functional Mobility and Active Lifestyles

Chapter 3

Community-Based Exercise for Health and Performance

Musa L. Mathunjwa, Senzelwe Mazibuko, Dimitar Avramov and Mukoma G. Gudani

Abstract

This chapter explores the physiological mechanisms and performance of community-based exercise interventions, reframing them as transformative tools for enhancing health in underserved and rural populations. As noncommunicable diseases (NCDs) such as hypertension, diabetes, and obesity rise due to sedentary lifestyles and limited healthcare access, the chapter demonstrates how culturally responsive physical activity programs can effectively prevent and manage these conditions. Bridging health, training, and technology, the discussion focuses on South African rural communities, advocating for group-based aerobic and resistance training models adapted to local realities. It critically reviews participation barriers, including infrastructural constraints and socio-economic pressures, while proposing feasible solutions such as peer-led sessions, the involvement of community health workers, and the inclusion of indigenous games to foster cultural resonance. Furthermore, the role of mobile technology and wearable devices is examined as a scalable method for monitoring progress, maintaining motivation, and ensuring program sustainability. By centering communities in the design of interventions, the chapter proposes a participatory, inclusive model that empowers individuals and fosters long-term behavioral change. These insights highlight the potential of community-based physical activity programs to rectify health disparities, improve quality of life, and support national public health objectives. This is particularly vital in resource-constrained environments where traditional healthcare provision is often inadequate.

Keywords: community-based exercise, physical activity, non-communicable diseases (NCDs), health promotion, rural populations, group training

1. Introduction

Community-based exercise programs are physical activity interventions designed to autonomously provide the intervention into local settings (community centers, schools, churches, parks, or clinics) [1]. Such programs tend to be based on the specific requirements, cultural values, and health issues of particular groups, especially underserved or rural people. They focus on inclusivity, accessibility, and sustainability, which are the vital features of managing an increased level of non-communicable diseases (NCDs) worldwide, including cardiovascular disease, diabetes, and obesity [2].

The fact that localized interventions in the field of public health are crucial because they make the communities active participants in the health and wellness process [3, 4]. In contrast to the top-down health promotion approaches, members of the community are active participants of those approaches in the form of community-based exercise programs. They enable individuals to empower by means of providing them with culturally appropriate, low cost, environmentally supportive physical activities [5]. These include the walking group in a township, the dance fitness class in a rural hall, and the structured indigenous games for youth that not only boost physical well-being but also mental and social health [5, 6].

It has been found out that such interventions enhance the compliance to exercises, lower medical bills and enhance better community cohesion. The research in Africa demonstrates encouraging results, such as decreased body mass index (BMI), the decreasing blood pressure levels, and enhanced quality of life in participants [7]. In addition, local physical activity programs play a central role in the environment where there are no facilities to get healthcare services [8, 9]. They also bridge the gap through use of local resources, peer support, which is quite essential in the modification of health behavior [10].

As the burden of NCDs in the world continues to shift towards low- and middle-income countries, interventions that are of interest and may be scaled up and sustained may include community-based exercise [11]. The policymakers and the professional communities of the public health practitioners are now beginning to realize their role in the promotion of health equity and physical literacy and in advancing the health outcomes of the community level [12].

2. Theoretical underpinnings

The promotion of physical activity cannot be external outside the theoretical framework multi-layered approach, at least in the fight against the non-communicable diseases (NCDs) [13]. These three primary frameworks which are included in this chapter include Social Ecological Model (SEM), Guide I Exercise Physiology, and Behavioral Change Models [14].

2.1 Social ecology model

The SEM provides a multidimensional framework in terms of which the way individual behaviors are shaped by multiple layers is determined, such as, intrapersonal, interpersonal, community, organizational, and policy levels [15]. It focuses on the connection between individuals and their social and physical environment to support the notion that powerful interventions must be made not only on the level of motivation of people but on the level of quality of environments and good policies [16]. As an illustration, one can enhance the engagement in physical activity particularly among the underserved communities like it is the case with rural communities through community integration, culturally relevant programming, as well as the accessibility of safe recreational spots [17, 18].

2.2 Macroergonomics principles

A community-based exercise programme cannot be designed and executed merely by giving a list of activities. It is the use of the basic concepts of exercise physiology overload, specificity, progression, and reversibility in a manner that can be comprehended and maintained by an ordinary person. These principles are not in the abstract sense, but are the natural reactions of the body to physical activity and long-term adaptation [19]. In practice, they result in meaningful health benefits and prevent non-communicable diseases (NCDs) in communities (World Health Organization) [20]. During acute physiologic reactions, the body instantly adapts to the new demands. The heart works harder and faster to deliver oxygenated blood to working muscles. At the same time, the lungs accelerate ventilation, which increases oxygen uptake to support energy needs [21]. To maintain activity, muscles stimulate more fibers, especially those that are able to generate more force. These are the short-term changes that can be predicted, and they happen whenever an individual takes a workout. They are temporary, but serve as the impulse to more profound, permanent adaptations when the activity is repeated regularly [22].

2.2.1 Chronic physiological adaptations

These acute responses become the long-term benefits with regular training. The heart works harder and more efficiently and expels more blood with each beat and reduces heart rate in rest [23]. This results in better stamina and less energy consumption in day-to-day activity. The density of the capillaries surrounding the muscles is enhanced, which assists in supplying oxygen and other nutrients to the muscles and eliminating wastes.

Regarding metabolic mechanisms, exercise optimizes energy, and better insulin sensitivity reduces the risk of type 2 diabetes [24]. The density of mitochondria in the muscle cells increases, allowing muscle cells to sustain longer physical activity with reduced fatigue. This makes the body an effective fat burner too and stores carbohydrates to be used in higher-intensity activities [25]. Resistance training also enhances neuromuscular coordination and muscle strength and increases balance and injury resilience, particularly in older adults [26].

2.2.2 Connecting principles to community programmes

These principles are applied successfully to provide beneficial community-based interventions. Overload is necessary to ensure that the body is sufficiently challenged to promote adaptation, whereas specificity is necessary to ensure that training is specific to desired results (e.g., walking to build endurance, resistance training to build strength). Progression emphasizes that, to prevent stagnation and injury, training load must be slowly increased, and reversibility cautions that without training, a person may start moving backward [27]. As an example, a walking group might start with small, easily manageable distances and slowly speed up and expand. Resistance training can begin with bodyweight exercises, and then the use of elastic bands and home objects. Notably, these programmes need to be welcoming and flexible enough to overcome age, health condition, and fitness level differences [28]. In this way, they establish convenient channels through which people can maintain healthy lifestyles and minimize the risks of NCDs in the community.

2.3 Principles of behavioral change

Designing an effective exercise program requires more than just understanding physiology; it requires an understanding of people. The true challenge lies not in initiating change, but in sustaining it. This is where behavioral change theories become indispensable, transforming a short-term regimen into a lasting lifestyle [29].

While physiology explains how the body adapts, behavioral science explores why people choose to engage and persist. Central to this is the concept of self-efficacy – an individual's belief in their own capability. By setting small, achievable goals, programs can build this confidence, creating a powerful internal motivator for continued participation 29. This internal drive is amplified by social support. Group activities foster a profound sense of community and shared identity, directly countering the isolation and lack of motivation that often derail progress [30].

Modern technology, such as wearable devices, complements these principles by providing immediate feedback, a core tenet of the Transtheoretical Model of Change. This model recognizes that individuals progress through distinct stages when adopting new behaviors, from contemplation to maintenance, and effective support must be tailored to each phase [31, 32].

The success of this holistic approach is evident in real-world applications. A 12-week indigenous dance program not only enhanced cultural connection but also delivered an average 8% increase in aerobic capacity [33]. Similarly, a community-led strength initiative using locally sourced materials achieved a remarkable 25% average gain in upper body strength [34].

These examples demonstrate that, by marrying physiological rigor with behavioral insight, community programs can transcend basic health benefits. They become empowering ecosystems that build both fitness and belief, proving that sustainable change is ultimately a human journey [35, 36].

2.4 Technological integration and physiological monitoring

The use of technology in community-based exercise programs offers a practical and scalable way to connect training principles with real-time physiological outcomes [37]. Instead of relying only on self-reports or occasional assessments which can be time-consuming and sometimes unreliable digital tools now make it possible to collect accurate, continuous data that helps design better programs and track individual progress [38]. Wearable devices such as Fitbit or chest-strap monitors can capture heart rate (HR), heart rate variability (HRV), and calories burned, allowing community programs to monitor changes in participants' bodies as they happen [39]. For example, HRV provides an easy, non-invasive way to look at how the autonomic nervous system is functioning, making it a useful indicator of recovery and training load [40]. If a participant's HRV starts to drop, it can signal that they are overtraining or not recovering well, giving program leaders a chance to adjust the exercises before problems arise [41]. Beyond monitoring heart rate, smartphones and GPS-enabled devices can track external workload factors [42]. GPS data, for instance, can measure distance, speed, and pace during aerobic activities, offering a clear picture of how intense and how long a training session is [43]. Smartwatches and fitness trackers often use accelerometers, which measure movement patterns and provide an estimate of total daily activity, energy expenditure, and adherence to the program [44]. All these data can then be shared with community health workers or program leaders, who can use it to give participants personalized feedback and motivational support [45].

This kind of feedback helps individuals see how their effort directly influences their health markers, boosting both confidence and commitment to the program [46]. In this way, technology transforms exercise programs from being static and directive into dynamic, adaptive, and data-driven interventions that respond to the unique needs of each participant [47].

2.5 Future research directions: Longitudinal and comparative studies

For these programs to influence public health policy and demonstrate their full potential, future studies need to use more rigorous research designs [48]. One important step would be conducting randomized controlled trials that compare the effects of culturally relevant activities, like indigenous games, with more traditional exercise methods such as high-intensity interval training (HIIT) or resistance training (RT) [49]. These studies should run for at least 6 to 12 months, so that researchers can measure long-term physiological changes and patterns of adherence [50]. For example, randomized trials could track outcomes such as VO_2max, muscular strength, and metabolic health markers when comparing indigenous games to HIIT or resistance training over this period [51]. The results would provide strong evidence to guide public health policy while highlighting how culturally adapted exercise programs can achieve meaningful health improvements, especially in communities with limited resources [52].

Together, these models guide the development of holistic, culturally sensitive, and sustainable interventions to promote physical activity and mitigate the risk of NCDs.

2.5.1 Integrated approach

Combining SEM, physiology, and behavior change theories enables the design of holistic and sustainable community-based programs:

SEM level	Theoretical component(s)	Application strategy	References
Individual	Transtheoretical Model (TTM); Health Belief Model (HBM)	Develop personalized health messaging aligned with individuals' stages of change; build self-efficacy and highlight perceived benefits.	[53]
Interpersonal	Social Cognitive Theory (SCT); Social Ecological Model (SEM)	Strengthen social support through peer-led activities, role modeling, and community-based learning within indigenous game settings.	[54]
Organizational/ community	Social Ecological Model (SEM); Principles of Exercise Physiology	Provide culturally responsive physical activity programs using indigenous games, ensuring safe environments and progressive challenges.	[6]
Policy/ environment	Public Health Frameworks; SEM; HBM	Advocate for infrastructure development (e.g., communal game spaces) and policy reforms to integrate indigenous games into public health.	[55]

Table 1.
Multi-level theoretical and application framework for promoting indigenous games and physical activity.

Table 1 demonstrates an Integrated Theoretical Model of Community-Based NCD Interventions that entails the combination of physiological, behavioral change and socio-environmental frameworks. This correlation makes the health initiatives effective and culturally based, thereby enhancing the participation and ultimate concentration. The model promotes the use of holistic interventions in the design, thereby promoting the aspect of community ownership, sustainability, and the efficacy of the NCD prevention and management efforts.

3. Exercise health benefits of community-based

Community-based exercise interventions are a method that is highly connected to culture and highly accessible to apply in special populations with limited resources (i.e., underserved or rural).

3.1 Non-communicable diseases (NCDs) reform

Regular physical activities in the community programs have revealed impressive results on risk factors of cancer, type 2 diabetes, hypertension, and obesity. On the basis of the data of the Indigenous-led intervention and meta-analysis, large effect is found on the parameters of blood pressure, level of HbA1c, and resting heart rate [18, 56]. After 8 weeks of aerobics intervention, an 8 percent increase in VO2 max was found and a systolic and diastolic blood pressure was considerably lowered [56].

3.2 Improved cardiovascular and muscular systems

Aerobic machinery and strength of muscles can also be enhanced using the combination of training programmes of damn exercises like circuit training and local games, in this case kgati (jump rope) [57]. In four decades, cardiovascular mortality in North Karelia Project in Finland went down by 82 per cent since it embraced a holistic solution where the whole lot of community members got the exercise [56]. The same fitness benefits have also been determined in the similar rural settings, which have again provided the evidence of universality of these programs [5, 18, 56].

3.3 Psychological and social benefits

Besides the physical advantages it attracts, community-based exercise has a psychological and social fortification nature [57]. The individuals who participated in Indigenous wellness activities showed the reduction of stress levels, positive mood, and increased community relationships [58]. The issue of cultural identity and emotional resilience through the traditional games and dancing is also an important aspect in the struggle against social isolation and adherence increment in the case of populations that are limited on resources [59].

Overall, circuit-type, indigenous games type, and culturally specific walking capital exercising programs are very appealing in their health implications in community-based exercise programs [60]. These are healthier hearts, and it cuts down the risk of NCD, strengthened mental health, and fortified social integration.

The evidence is highly in favor of including culturally specific activities into the health promotion strategies of the rural areas and especially resource-poor areas [61].

4. The administration of exercises in the community

4.1 Needs assessment, and community engagement

The introduction of an effective community-based exercise-based intervention must begin with the implementation of a thorough needs assessment in which the local needs and preferences should reflect on the developed program [62]. This will involve focus groups, merger interviews, and consult with the local leaders, health workers, and prospective participants. In a further explanation on what [63] has indicated, incorporating the stakeholders at a relatively early period into the process implies they can help to identify the barriers, which may include safety concerns, in the process and too good to mention is that it helps to make the process culturally appropriate [63]. One of them is the ownership of co-creation of the intervention by the formation of community advisory committee that assists in the sustainability of the intervention.

4.2 Kind of exercises

The community-based interventions mostly combine applied aerobic, resistance, and flexibility/mobility parts: Aerobic exercises: walking groups, culturally-relevant dance fitness classes, jump-rope (skipping) circles are the most effective means of offering cardiovascular health, even as they promote social affiliations [64]. In an illustration, there is positive improvement of VO 2 max, cardiovascular risk factors in type 2 diabetic severities in low cost community-based walking associations [65]. Bodyweight circuits and elastic-band workouts offer progressive strength work. The studies show that community-based resistance training is effective to enhance the cardiometabolic risk and the muscle strength along with the mature-aged individuals [56, 66]. Flexibility and mobility: Combinations of heavy stretching routines and Yoga-like flowing help to improve the ROM and the joint health, compensating the aerobic and resistance trainings.

4.3 Flow and structure of the session

Sessions are discussed in accordance with the program models to occur 3–5 days a week with a duration of 45–70 minutes each time [67]. Every session will include a 5–10-minute warm-up, 20–30 minutes of low to moderate intensity aerobic exercise (50–70 percent heart rate max or rate of perception 11–14) followed by 20–30 minutes of resistance training (2–3 sets of 10–15 repetitions) and ending with a 5–10 minute cooldown and stretch [68]. It is followed by a periodical increment in the intensity of exercise or volume seeking. For example:

Weeks 1–4: Light intensity (walking, light bands).

Weeks 5–8: Brisk walking or being on the move, moderate resistance.

Weeks 9–12+: Increased volume, integrated agility drill, or complicated resistance exercises.

Such programs as 9-month diabetes intervention that comprised three times per week sessions showed impressive results on improving a walk test (+8%), a chair stand (+29%), and balance (+14%) [69], proving the importance of a consistent regime and different types of exercises.

4.4 Employing engagements and safety

The programs will be delivered in the form of classes organized in groups with the involvement of professional participation of community health workers or other trained health workers. It results in a very fundamental motivation and social support to adherence [70]. Furthermore, the sessions must be universal and adaptable and have alternative forms of modalities to suit various capabilities (e.g. seated exercises, less energetic substitutes). The programs should entail basic risk screen and continuous monitor that is accompanied by evaluation, including heart rate and RPE [71].

4.5 Long term sustainability

The programs should also include training of the community facilitators in as far as they would train to provide effects of sustainability, that is, local ownership. Community suitability and compatibility is also enhanced by anchoring sessions in already existing community facilities, community places of worship and community educational institutions [72]. Iterative development of sessions and refinements is presented in form of cycles of feedback supplied on surveys or groups of people reflecting on developments in aid to indicate direction [73]. Finally, the clear monitoring and evaluation-driven systems unite long-term financing and lifelong learning, including the pre- and post-health measurements and qualitative feedback.

5. Practical examples and indigenous games

5.1 Kgati

Community-based and culturally relevant physical activity results in community-based and culturally significant exercise by means of a Kgati (jump rope) Wellness Program led by females, which yoga enthusiasts assert enhances body compositions, endurance, and moods in Vhembe District [74]. This just resonates with the overall tendency in the rural area in KwaZulu Natal whereby organized physical activities like walking programs or indigenous games have resulted in good health outcomes among the local people. Consider the case of Ingwavuma (neighboring uMkhanyakude District): the adults averaged over 900 minutes of physical activity per week that is tremendously up at the risk of cardiovascular diseases [75].

5.2 Morabaraba: A motion of brain and body interaction of the seniors

The Morabaraba Move game is an initiative that brings together the elderly community in the rural communities to be the members of the monthly get-togethers involving the traditional game of Morabaraba [76] and the recreational activity of taking the walks. The mental process – the tactics of Morabaraba – is not the only process activated during this two-dimensional form of exercise but a healthy condition of the heart as well, which is synonymous with holistic intervention brought to nursing homes, the implementation of which led to a better mood and mobility of the residents [77].

5.3 Keeping fit in school-KwaZulu Natal

There is a creative program introduced before and after classes in one of the high schools in a rural area in KwaZulu Natal which incorporates music, indigenous dance, and group cardiovascular circuit [78]. This program significantly reduced the degree of sedentary behavior among adolescents, indicative of the findings of the research performed on a provincial basis in terms that the degree of inactivity is shocking and the presence of such culturally integrated interventions have the potential of rectifying the scenario [79, 80].

6. Implementation barriers

6.1 Psycholinguistics socioeconomic and cultural factors

The socioeconomic status is another factor that hinders the outreach of the NCD programs, and it has been a continuing issue among the poor and rural populations. Economics disadvantages the economic players as they gain limited access to routine care, drugs, and sessions of programs due to economic need [53]. To provide an example, a study conducted in Ethiopia and Bangladesh reports that individuals tend to skip visits to the clinic due to the costs of traveling and treatment costs [54]. Cultural norms and gender roles add further problems to these: there is a social stigma against sickness or using medical services otherwise, negative attitudes towards using medical services in the first place, which will push women and other disadvantaged populations away using preventative services [54].

6.2 Infrastructure and environment related problem

Another vital infrastructure also in the provision of effective interventions against NCD is essential. The available equipment like the BP machine, glucometers, as well as a consultation room among others are not suitable or do not exist in most of the primary care and community facilities, talk less of a consultation room [81]. Furthermore, the features of physical environment lacking in safety or proper physical settings like poor road network, poorly located health facilities and lack of transportation, especially during times of bad weather, are also a significant obstacle towards access [82].

6.3 Training and human resources

Lastly, shortage of human resources and poor training of the community health workers (CHWs) proves to be one more factor that limits the success of the NCD programs. The overworked staff will not be able to give high-quality interventions, and, moreover, the high turnover is a disaster to the program continuity [83]. CHWs within a given setting remain unqualified to integrate NCD provisions or consult patients well, and this substantiates the need of well-disciplined and supervised capacity-building systems [84].

7. Widespread usage of technological integration in community exercise

7.1 SMS programs and mobile applications

A possibility of mobile use, such as WhatsApp and SMS programs, to deliver the workouts, enhance accountability, and increase participation has been there. To illustrate, the 10-week WhatsApp-based intervention on elderly people improved the aerobic capacity and reduced blood pressure yet at a weaker magnitude in comparison with face-to-face training [85]. Further, SMS-based systems in which there is a daily record of the number of steps also improves the involvement of the rural women because of encouragement and motivation [86].

7.2 Wearable devices

Heart rate monitors and other pedometers enhance motivation and self-monitoring group-based activities. Wearable monitors have demonstrated the production of significant improvements in physical activity daily steps, MVPA, and quality of life in people with chronic diseases [87]. Among the rural older adults, Fitbit products were deemed suitable and acceptable, although a few users required assistance with the set up [88, 89]. Additional motivation of participants, especially less active ones, is created through elements of gamification where participants compete to raise the number of steps (step competition) or earn a position on the leaderboard [65].

7.3 Barriers to technology adoption

Though its usage is potentially beneficial, there are a lot of challenges in its adoption in the rural communities. Usage can be restricted by device access, charging, and literacy. Most of the interventions will need personnel on site to run machines and the network connection is also slow in streaming if any. Adherence also is affected by battery life and the accuracy of the devices [90].

8. Monitoring and evaluation

In community-based settings, monitoring and evaluation (M&E) is essential in the progress, and the effectiveness of interventions should focus on non-communicable diseases (NCDs). Sound M&E systems will make the interventions evidence-based, flexible, and sustainable in the long run [91].

8.1 Performance metrics

Motivating variables include objective measures such as of physical changes and functional health enhances, including 6-Minute Walk Test (6MWT), Sit-to-Stand Test, BMI, and Resting Heart Rate, are used to track the physical adaption and functional health outcomes [92]. Such instruments provide quality information on cardiorespiratory endurance, muscular strength, and body composition [93]. Regular re-evaluation enables altering an exercise program and pointing at the change in physical health in the long-term perspective [94].

8.2 The health indicators

Examples of physiological measurements that identify a cardiometabolic risk include blood pressure, fasting glucose, and waist measurements after a 10-week aerobic exercise program (Tae-bo) were also observed [56]. These indicators are comparable to foreign standards of NCD surveillance [95], and the regular review helps to detect these illnesses early, make the necessary medical referrals in a timely manner, and show success or failure of the intervention measures.

8.3 Qualitative answer

The focus groups, surveys, and personal journals are the qualitative tools that are utilized the compensation for the quantitative measures. These tools provide insight into the experience, perceived advantages, and major challenges of the participants. The mixed-methods evaluation triangulates the data, thereby ensuring that the health outcomes together with the voice of the participants will synergize, so as to affect the enhancement of the programs [96].

9. Partners and partnership appeals to the policy

The evolution of sustainable measures during prevention of non-communicable diseases (NCDs) and improvement of physical activity among the people in the rural areas require policy-reinforced involvement with policy as well as collaborations at the local level. This section outlines strategic pathways to the strengthening of partnership.

9.1 Community and health partnership

Having the experience of the available health infrastructure for any sport intervention can maximize the chances of early diagnosis and successful referrals. This can be seen in the case of routine cardiovascular medical check-up with the local district medical centers, and this can be combined with active involvement with the native as well as the organized physical exercise programs [97]. The most appropriate example is the community-based screening campaigns that have been effectively introduced by the Department of Health in KwaZulu-Natal, Mpumalanga and Free State provinces [98]. The building of referral networks between the community-based exercise programs and the local health facilities will be useful in terms of delivering the participants with the follow-up care they need and helping solve the problems of people health surveillance and the prevention of the NCD risk.

9.2 Role of municipalities and NGOs

To obtain optimal coverage, especially in rural under-serviced surroundings, municipalities should develop local infrastructures such as sports centers, walking tracks, and other exercising parks at community level premises [99]. The local governments under the mandate of SALGA according to Section 152 of the Constitution are empowered to pursue social development like the sport infrastructure [100]. Further, the NGO, Africa AHEAD, and Witkoppen Clinic direct us on how to carry out health promotion in the community-engaged organization [101]. The enhanced cooperation between the municipal and the NGOs would also be one of the methods to speed up the resources and quality of the services offered [102].

9.3 The National Health and Sport Strategies

Community programmes should also correspond to the national policy regarding mass participation and active lifestyles [12, 18, 103]. The ability of sport to promote health gains strength as countries incorporate physical activity agenda in NCD prevention plans. Action points in coordination of health, education, transport, and sports areas have to be established according to the general suggestion of the WHO. Accountability, resource planning and sustainable community health outcomes are served by such coordinated plans [4, 104–106].

10. Research gaps and future directions

The suitability and sustainability of the effect of rural non-communicable disease (NCD) intervention needs to be determined, and consequently, longitudinal study is one of the future research activities. Reactions on gender grounds particularly on women having social and financial problems should be further studied to have specific and more effective treatment procedures. In addition, realization of low cost digital health gadgets, that is, mHealth and telehealth services are significant to enable round the clock NCD learning and monitoring in the event and locations which do not have the digital development infrastructure foundation. Finally, the adherence of current traditional health beliefs is one of the sensitive parts of the assessment, which may be used to increase community-based interventions and participation. These gaps will be reduced to contribute to the enhancement of the equitability, sustainability, and effectiveness of NCD plans among the rural populations.

11. Conclusion

Exercise programming through the community is an effective means of promoting health among rural and underserved. Such programs are based on both exercise science and behavioral psychology, and culturally based activities are used to improve health variables such as blood pressure, glucose levels, and physical fitness. They encourage motivation and adherence through the integration of such principles of gaining progressive overload and social support. Technology such as mobile apps and wearable monitors can assist and customize assistance to personal requirements. The involvement of community leaders, health workers, and fitness professionals in paired work will make sure that the programs will be localized accordingly. Leadership is, however, what sustains resources, personnel training, and community ownership in the long term.

Conflict of interest

The authors declare no conflict of interest.

DOI: http://dx.doi.org/10.5772/intechopen.1014631

Author details

Musa L. Mathunjwa[1*], Senzelwe Mazibuko[2], Dimitar Avramov[3]
and Mukoma G. Gudani[4]

1 University of Zululand, KwaDlangezwa, South Africa

2 Senzelwisihe Rehabilitation Hospital, Empangeni, South Africa

3 National Sports Academy, University of Bulgaria, Sofia, Bulgaria

4 Department of Biokinetics, Recreation and Sports Science, University of Venda, Thohoyandou, South Africa

*Address all correspondence to: mathunjwam@unizulu.ac.za

References

[1] Gavin JP, Holt LC, Muckelt PE, Sadler E, McDonough S, Barker M. Maintaining physical activity in people with long-term conditions following engagement in physical activity referral schemes: Barriers, enablers, and intervention strategies. The International Journal of Behavioral Nutrition and Physical Activity. 2025;**22**:102. DOI: 10.1186/s12966-025-01802-y

[2] Khan B. The role of lifestyle interventions in preventing and managing non-communicable diseases. Non-Communicable Diseases and Care. 2025;**2**(1):50-60. DOI: 10.59613/global.v2i1.75

[3] Shaikh M, Birajdar F. Ensuring purity and health: A comprehensive study of water quality testing labs in Solapur district for community well-being. International Journal of Innovative Science and Research Technology. 2024;**9**(1):271-281. DOI: 10.5281/zenodo.10521637

[4] Mathunjwa ML, Nduduzo SM, Schoeman H, Linda N, Linda N, Nkwanyana S, et al. The need for community-centered intervention strategies on promoting health living in individuals with type 2 diabetes mellitus (T2DM) and human immunodeficiency virus (HIV) in South Africa. Medical Research Archives. 2024;**12**(12):1-8. DOI: 10.18103/mra.v12i12.5938

[5] Dube A, Shaw I, Mathunjwa ML, Shaw BS. Impact of traditional dance and games on cardiovascular health: A scoping review of outcomes across diverse low-and middle-income countries. International Journal of Environmental Research and Public Health. 2025;**22**(3):440. DOI: 10.3390/ijerph22030440

[6] Sakala M. Indigenous Games as Part of School-Based Physical Activity Delivery Programmes: Prospects for Optimum Implementation for Primary School Learners' Holistic Health Outcomes. South Africa: University of Johannesburg; 2023. Available from: https://hdl.handle.net/10210/505174

[7] Shandu NM, Mathunjwa ML, Shaw I, Shaw BS. Exercise effects on health-related quality of life (HRQOL), muscular function, cardiorespiratory function, and body composition in smokers: A narrative review. International Journal of Environmental Research and Public Health. 2023;**20**(19):6813. DOI: 10.3390/ijerph20196813

[8] Zhong J, Liu W, Niu B, Lin X, Deng Y. Role of built environments on physical activity and health promotion: A review and policy insights. Frontiers in Public Health. 2022;**12**(10):950348

[9] Cipta DA, Andoko D, Theja A, Utama AV, Hendrik H, William DG, et al. Culturally sensitive patient-centered healthcare: A focus on health behavior modification in low and middle-income nations—Insights from Indonesia. Frontiers in Medicine. 2024;**12**(11):1353037. DOI: 10.3389/fpubh.2022.950348

[10] Abrahams N, Khodabakhsh S, Toumpakari Z, Marais F, Lambert EV, Foster C. Using social networks to scale up and sustain community-based programmes to improve physical activity and diet in low-income and middle-income countries: A scoping review. International Journal of Behavioral Nutrition and Physical Activity. 2023;**20**(1):8. DOI: 10.1186/s12966-023-01412-6

[11] Shaw I, Mathunjwa ML, Shaw BS. Physical activity and health promotion: A public health imperative. In: Health Promotion-Principles and Approaches. London, UK: IntechOpen; 2023. p. 14. DOI: 10.5772/intechopen.111927

[12] Ominyi J, Clifton A, Nwedu A. Understanding physical activity participation among underserved women: A mixed-methods cross sectional study using an ecological framework. BMC Public Health. 2025;**25**(1):2178. DOI: 10.1186/s12889-025-23189-y

[13] Johannes C, Roman N. Applying the social ecological model to explore physical activity levels and psychosocial factors among undergraduate university students: A narrative literature review. The Open Public Health Journal. 2025;**18**(1):1-15. DOI: 10.2174/0118749445392277250428114135

[14] Saglam MH, Goktenturk T, Demir I, Yazıcı E. Environmental factors for the advancement of teachers' self-efficacy in professional development. Journal of Intelligence. 2023;**11**(2):28. DOI: 10.3390/jintelligence11020028

[15] Kemp SP, Whittaker JK, Tracy EM. Person-Environment Practice: Social Ecology of Interpersonal Helping. Taylor & Francis; 2024. p. 1. DOI: 10.4324/9781003571865

[16] Bantham A, Ross SE, Sebastião E, Hall G. Overcoming barriers to physical activity in underserved populations. Progress in Cardiovascular Diseases. 2021;**1**(64):64-71. DOI: 10.1016/j.pcad.2020.11.002

[17] Mathunjwa M, Shaw I, Moran J, Sandercock GR, Brown GA, Shaw BS. Implementation of a community-based mind–body (Tae-Bo) physical activity programme on health-related physical fitness in rural black overweight and obese women with manifest risk factors for multimorbidity. International Journal of Environmental Research and Public Health. 2023;**20**(15):1-17. DOI: 10.3390/ijerph20156463

[18] Hersman RK, Younis R, Farabaugh B, Goldblum B, Reddie A. Under the Nuclear Shadow: Situational Awareness Technology and Crisis Decisionmaking. Bloomsbury Publishing PLC; 2021. p. 15. DOI: 10.15868/SOCIALSECTOR.39937

[19] Kelly LE. Adapted Physical Education National Standards. Champaign, Switzerland: Human Kinetics Publishers; 2020

[20] World Health Organization. Tackling NCDs: Best Buys and Other Recommended Interventions for the Prevention and Control of Noncommunicable Diseases. Geneva, Switzerland: World Health Organization; 2024

[21] Ferretti G, Fagoni N, Taboni A, Vinetti G, di Prampero PE. A century of exercise physiology: Key concepts on coupling respiratory oxygen flow to muscle energy demand during exercise. European Journal of Applied Physiology. 2022;**122**(6):1317-1365

[22] Maloof M. The Spark Factor: The Secret to Supercharging Energy, Becoming Resilient and Feeling Better than Ever. UK: Hachette; 2023

[23] Akram M. Heart rate recovery (HRR). Journal of Microbes and Research. 2024;**3**(1):2836-2187

[24] Małkowska P. Positive effects of physical activity on insulin signaling. Current Issues in Molecular Biology. 2024;**46**(6):5467-5487. DOI: 10.3390/cimb46060327

[25] Prins PJ, Noakes TD, Buga A, D'Agostino DP, Volek JS, Buxton JD, et al. Low and high carbohydrate isocaloric diets on performance, fat oxidation, glucose and cardiometabolic health in middle-aged males. Frontiers in Nutrition. 2023;**10**:1084021. DOI: 10.3389/fnut.2023.1084021

[26] Zhong YJ, Meng Q, Su CH. Mechanism-driven strategies for reducing fall risk in the elderly: A multidisciplinary review of exercise interventions. Healthcare. 2024;**12**(23):2394. DOI: 10.3390/healthcare12232394

[27] Rodríguez S, Suarez-Cuervo AN, León-Prieto C. Exercise progressions and regressions in sports training and rehabilitation. Journal of Bodywork and Movement Therapies. 2024;**40**:1879-1889. DOI: 10.1016/j.jbmt.2024.10.026

[28] Ginis KAM, van der Ploeg HP, Foster C, Lai B, McBride CB, Ng K, et al. Participation of people living with disabilities in physical activity: A global perspective. The Lancet. 2021;**398**(10298):443-455. DOI: 10.1016/S0140-6736(21)01164-8

[29] Hasanain B. The role of ergonomic and human factors in sustainable manufacturing: A review. Machines. 2024;**12**(3):159. DOI: 10.3390/machines12030159

[30] Mina HA. Motivational Peer Influence on Behavior Change in Undergraduates: A Phenomenological Study. London, UK: Taylor & Francis; 2025. Available from: https://digitalcommons.liberty.edu/doctoral/7108

[31] DiClemente CC, Graydon MM. 10 changing behavior using the transtheoretical model. In: The Handbook of Behavior Change. Burlington, MA: Jones & Bartlett Learning; 2020. p. 136. DOI: 10.1017/9781108677318.010

[32] Caffarella DL. Describing clients' progress through the transtheoretical model stages of change [doctoral dissertation]. Phoenix, AZ: Grand Canyon University; 2025

[33] Mesfin AA. Effects of aerobic exercise on selected health related physical fitness of students in Kara Magane Secondary School, Ginnir Wereda, East Bale Oromiya Regional State, Ethiopia [doctoral dissertation]. Haramaya, Ethiopia: Haramaya University; 2022

[34] Sigvaldsen E, Loturco I, Larsen F, Bruusgaard J, Kalhovde JM, Haugen T. Validity and reliability of upper body push and pull tests to determine one-repetition maximum. PLoS One. 2023;**18**(7):e0288649. DOI: 10.1371/journal.pone.0288649

[35] Garner CT. Utilizing community capitals to revitalize rural communities through extension programming [doctoral dissertation]. Athens, GA: University of Georgia; 2024

[36] Swargiary K. Health Education: Foundations, Strategies, and Innovations. US: EdTech Research Association; 2024

[37] Moon K, Hong JI, Kim J. Data-driven smart living lab: Enhancing community-based rehabilitation and sports participation for individuals with disabilities. In: International Sports Analytics Conference and Exhibition. Springer Nature Switzerland: Cham; 2024. pp. 137-148

[38] Edwards Q, Idoko B, Idoko JE, Ejembi EV, Onuh EP. Remote monitoring of social behavior in children with

autism: The role of digital phenotyping in public programs. Journal of Autism and Developmental Disorders. 2024;**21**(02):164-203. DOI: 10.30574/gscarr.2024.21.2.0413

[39] Alugubelli N, Abuissa H, Roka A. Wearable devices for remote monitoring of heart rate and heart rate variability—What we know and what is coming. Sensors. 2022;**22**(22):8903. DOI: 10.3390/s22228903

[40] Stephenson MD, Thompson AG, Merrigan JJ, Stone JD, Hagen JA. Applying heart rate variability to monitor health and performance in tactical personnel: A narrative review. International Journal of Environmental Research and Public Health. 2021;**18**(15):8143. DOI: 10.3390/ijerph18158143

[41] Roa JA. The Science of Peak Sports Performance: A Guide to the Assessment, Control, and Monitoring of Training. Cham, Switzerland: Springer Nature; 2024

[42] Farooq MS, Sohail OO, Abid A, Rasheed S. A survey on the role of iot in agriculture for the implementation of smart livestock environment. IEEE Access. 2022;**10**:9483-9505. DOI: 10.1109/ACCESS.2022.3166634

[43] Torres-Ronda L, Beanland E, Whitehead S, Sweeting A, Clubb J. Tracking systems in team sports: A narrative review of applications of the data and sport specific analysis. Sports Medicine-Open. 2022;**8**(1):15. DOI: 10.1186/s40798-022-00408-z

[44] Straczkiewicz M, Huang EJ, Onnela JP. A "one-size-fits-most" walking recognition method for smartphones, smartwatches, and wearable accelerometers. npj Digital Medicine. 2023;**6**(1):29

[45] Majee W, Anakwe A, Johnson L, Rhoda A, Frantz J, Schopp L. A self-management training intervention: Perceptions and practices of community health workers in South Africa. Health Promotion Practice. 2020;**21**(6):983-992. DOI: 10.1177/1524839918820038

[46] Bandura A. Cultivate self-efficacy for personal and organizational effectiveness. In: Principles of Organizational Behavior: The Handbook of Evidence-Based Management. 3rd ed. Champaign, IL: Human Kinetics; 2023. pp. 113-135. DOI: 10.1002/9781394320769.ch6

[47] Addolorato S. Can wearable and digital technologies augment business-to-consumer data driven outcomes in health and fitness industry? Sport i Turystyka. 2025;**8**(1):161-175. DOI: 10.16926/sit.2025.01.08

[48] Masood S, Kothari A, Regan S. The use of research in public health policy: A systematic review. Evidence & Policy. 2020;**16**(1):7-43. DOI: 10.1332/174426418X15193814624487

[49] Harris N, Warbrick I, Fleming T, Borotkanics R, Atkins D, Lubans D. Impact of high-intensity interval training including indigenous narratives on adolescents' mental health: A cluster-randomised controlled trial. Australian and New Zealand Journal of Public Health. 2022;**46**(6):794-799. DOI: 10.1111/1753-6405.13312

[50] Tang LM, Kay J. Harnessing long term physical activity data—How long-term trackers use data and how an adherence-based interface supports new insights. Proceedings of the ACM on Interactive, Mobile, Wearable and Ubiquitous Technologies. 2017;**1**(2):1-28. DOI: 10.1145/309009

[51] Moro T, Marcolin G, Bianco A, Bolzetta F, Berton L, Sergi G, et al. Effects of 6 weeks of traditional resistance training or high intensity interval resistance training on body composition, aerobic power and strength in healthy young subjects: A randomized parallel trial. International Journal of Environmental Research and Public Health. 2020;**17**(11):4093. DOI: 10.3390/ijerph17114093

[52] Bopp M. Physical Activity in Diverse Populations: Evidence and Practice. New York, NY, London, UK: Taylor & Francis; 2025. DOI: 10.4324/9781003474159

[53] Li H, Zhang W, Yan J. Physical activity and sedentary behavior among school-going adolescents in low-and middle-income countries: Insights from the global school-based health survey. PeerJ. 2024;**24**(12):e17097. DOI: 10.7717/peerj.17097

[54] Cindi L. Incorporating African indigenous knowledge systems into the basic education curriculum: Experiences from two schools in the Gauteng and KwaZulu-Natal Provinces, South Africa. London, UK: Taylor & Francis; 2024. Available from: http://hdl.handle.net/11660/11720

[55] Almansoori A, Al-Emran M, Shaalan K. Determinants of users' cybersecurity behavior in the metaverse: A deep learning-based hybrid SEM-ANN approach. International Journal of Human–Computer Interaction. 2024;**17**:1-8. DOI: 10.1080/10447318.2024.2440674

[56] Mathunjwa ML, Semple SJ, du Preez C. A 10-week aerobic exercise program reduces cardiometabolic disease risk in overweight/obese female African University students. Ethnicity & Disease. 2013;**23**(2):143-148. Available from: http://pubmed.ncbi.nlm.nih.gov/23530293/

[57] Dube MH. Effect of skipping rope on lower body strength, speed and cardiovascular endurance among U-15 male football Project Akaki Kality Sub-City, Addis Ababa, Ethiopia [doctoral dissertation]. Pretoria, South Africa: Haramaya University; 2024. Available from: http://ir.haramaya.edu.et//hru/handle/123456789/6862

[58] Alimam S. Building a Markov Model for Economic Evaluation of a Community-Based CVDs Prevention Program–Case North Karelia Project in Finland. Amsterdam, Netherlands: Elsevier; 2023. Available from: http://urn.fi/urn:nbn:fi:uef-20201018

[59] Hellison D, Martinek TJ, Wright P, Walsh D. Teaching Personal and Social Responsibility through Physical Activity. Sydney, Australia: Human Kinetics; 2025. p. 27. DOI: 10.5040/9781718208919

[60] Ahmed F, Zuk AM, Tsuji LJ. The impact of land-based physical activity interventions on self-reported health and well-being of indigenous adults: A systematic review. International Journal of Environmental Research and Public Health. 2021;**18**(13):7099. DOI: 10.3390/ijerph18137099

[61] Afolaranmi VB, Afolaranmi AO. Cultural revitalization through dance as a panacea for peacebuilding. Advanced Journal of Theatre and Film Studies. 2024;**2**(1):39-45. DOI: 10.57040/e4ywhy31

[62] Salameh AB. Early intervention among Jordanian youth at risk for T2DM to prevent disease onset and complications, through lifestyle change and self-efficacy [doctoral dissertation]. Thousand Oaks, CA: University of the Sunshine Coast; 2025

[63] Van Zyl C, Badenhorst M, Hanekom S, Heine M. Unravelling

'low-resource settings': A systematic scoping review with qualitative content analysis. BMJ Global Health. 2021;**6**(6):1-14. DOI: 10.1136/bmjgh-2021-005190

[64] Aravind G, Bashir K, Cameron JI, Bayley MT, Teasell RW, Howe JA, et al. What matters to program partners when implementing a community-based exercise program for people post-stroke? A theory-based qualitative study and cost analysis. Frontiers in Rehabilitation Sciences. 2023;**4**(4):1064206. DOI: 10.3389/fresc.2023.1064206

[65] Reyes DK. Employee merger perspectives: A qualitative study of social service nonprofits in Los Angeles County [doctoral dissertation]. Riverside, CA: California Baptist University; 2025. DOI: 10.1108/PR-06-2012-0096

[66] Bogataj Š, Pajek M, Kren A, Mesarič KK, Pajek J. Randomized controlled trial of intradialytic cognitive and physical training to enhance functional capacity. Kidney International Reports. 2024;**9**(7):2028-2036. DOI: 10.1016/j.ekir.2024.04.029

[67] Ungvari Z, Fazekas-Pongor V, Csiszar A, Kunutsor SK. The multifaceted benefits of walking for healthy aging: From blue zones to molecular mechanisms. Geroscience. 2023;**45**(6):3211-3239. DOI: 10.1007/s11357-023-00873-8

[68] Kang D, Park J, Eun SD. The efficacy of community-based exercise programs on circulating Irisin level, muscle strength, cardiorespiratory endurance, and body composition for ischemic stroke: A randomized controlled trial. Frontiers in Neurology. 2023;**29**(14):1187666. DOI: 10.3389/fneur.2023.1187666

[69] Atikumi N. Effect of long-duration aerobic exercises and exercise-scheduling on physiological and anthropometric health markers: A case study of a keep-fit club members in Accra, Ghana [doctoral dissertation]. Amsterdam, Netherlands: University of Cape Coast; 2024. Available from: http://hdl.handle.net/123456789/11130

[70] Staron A, Rybicki J, Rossouw A. Exercise training protocols. In: Exercise Programming for Cardiac Patients. Cham: Springer Nature Switzerland; 2025. pp. 61-99

[71] Sharma N, Chahal A, Balasubramanian K, Sanjeevi RR, Rai RH, Bansal N, et al. Effects of resistance training on muscular strength, endurance, body composition and functional performance among sarcopenic patients: A systematic review. Journal of Diabetes & Metabolic Disorders. 2023;**22**(2):1053-1071. DOI: 10.1007/s40200-023-01283-5

[72] Scott K, Beckham SW, Gross M, Pariyo G, Rao KD, Cometto G, et al. What do we know about community-based health worker programs? A systematic review of existing reviews on community health workers. Human Resources for Health. 2018;**16**(1):39. DOI: 10.1186/s12960-018-0304-x

[73] Gibson AL, Wagner DR, Heyward VH. Advanced Fitness Assessment and Exercise Prescription. Champaign, IL: Human Kinetics; 2024

[74] Glazier RA. Faith and Community: How Engagement Strengthens Members, Places of Worship, and Society. Vol. 5. Philadelphia, PA: Temple University Press; 2024

[75] Cennamo K, Kalk D. Real World Instructional Design: An Iterative Approach to Designing Learning Experiences. New York, NY: Routledge; 2019

[76] Chopra S. Niwh Yizt'iyh hilht'iz nets' eelh'iyh–"strengthening our bodies": The values and barriers to physical activity in remote and rural first Nations Communities in Northern British Columbia [doctoral dissertation]. Pretoria, South Africa: University of British Columbia; 2022. Available from: http://hdl.handle.net/2429/89044

[77] Chikafu H, Chimbari M. Hypertension care cascade in the Ingwavuma rural community, uMkhanyakude district, KwaZulu-Natal province of South Africa. PeerJ. 2021;**11**(9):e12372. DOI: 10.7717/peerj.12372

[78] Franco IB, Tracey J. Community capacity-building for sustainable development: Effectively striving towards achieving local community sustainability targets. International Journal of Sustainability in Higher Education. 2019;**20**(4):691-725. DOI: 10.1108/IJSHE-02-2019-0052

[79] Meeran S, Kodisang SM, Moila MM, Davids MN, Makokotlela MV. Ethnomathematics in intermediate phase: Reflections on the Morabaraba game as indigenous mathematical knowledge. African Journal of Research in Mathematics, Science and Technology Education. 2024;**28**(2):171-184. DOI: 10.1080/18117295.2024.2340095

[80] Zimu PM, Van Heerden HJ, Grace JM. Nyakaza-move-for-health: A culturally tailored physical activity intervention for adolescents in South Africa using the intervention mapping protocol. Journal of Primary Care & Community Health. 2024;**15**:21501319241278849. DOI: 10.3390/ijerph21060717

[81] Engdawork K, D'Ambruoso L, Hailu T, Yared M, Geletu GM, Baraki SG, et al. "Space to see the future"? A political economy analysis of child and adolescent mental health and well-being in Ethiopia including routes for change. Frontiers in Sociology. 2025;**9**:1488619. DOI: 10.3389/fsoc.2024.1488619

[82] Hasan MZ, Mehdi GG, Tisha KI, Rabbani MG, Ahmed MW, Paul S, et al. Costs of outpatient services at selected primary healthcare centers in Bangladesh: A cross-sectional study. PLoS One. 2025;**20**(1):e0317317. DOI: 10.1371/journal.pone.0317317

[83] Mulugeta TK, Kassa DH. Readiness of the primary health care units and associated factors for the management of hypertension and type II diabetes mellitus in Sidama, Ethiopia. PeerJ. 2022;**10**:e13797. DOI: 10.7717/peerj.13797

[84] Bonaccorsi G, Manzi F, Del Riccio M, Setola N, Naldi E, Milani C, et al. Impact of the built environment and the neighborhood in promoting the physical activity and the healthy aging in older people: An umbrella review. International Journal of Environmental Research and Public Health. 2020;**17**(17):6127. DOI: 10.3390/ijerph17176127

[85] Botiba A, Bakare D, Schlosser E. Revitalizing employee network and ensuring workforce stability. HMPI: Health Management, Policy & Innovation. 2024;**9**:1

[86] Rawal L, Jubayer S, Choudhury SR, Islam SM, Abdullah AS. Community health workers for non-communicable diseases prevention and control in Bangladesh: A qualitative study. Global Health Research and Policy. 2021;**6**(1):1. DOI: 10.1186/s41256-020-00182-z

[87] Muntaner-Mas A, Vidal-Conti J, Borras PA, Ortega FB, Palou P. Effects of a Whatsapp-delivered physical activity intervention to enhance health-related physical fitness components

and cardiovascular disease risk factors in older adults. The Journal of Sports Medicine and Physical Fitness. 2017;**57**(1-2):90-102. DOI: 10.23736/S0022-4707.16.05918-1

[88] Fjeldsoe BS, Miller YD, Marshall AL. MobileMums: A randomized controlled trial of an SMS-based physical activity intervention. Annals of Behavioral Medicine. 2010;**39**(2):101-111. DOI: 10.1007/s12160-010-9170-z

[89] Mathunjwa BM, Chen YF, Tsai TC, Hsu YL. A lifestyle monitoring system for older adults living independently using low-resolution smart meter data. Sensors. 2024;**24**(11):3662. DOI: 10.3390/s24113662

[90] Wiebe M, Mackay M, Krishnan R, Tian J, Larsson J, Modanloo S, et al. Feasibility characteristics of wrist-worn fitness trackers in health status monitoring for post-covid patients in remote and rural areas. PLOS Digital Health. 2024;**3**(8):e0000571. DOI: 10.1371/journal.pdig.0000571

[91] Park S, Kim S. Leaderboard design principles to enhance learning and motivation in a gamified educational environment: Development study. JMIR Serious Games. 2021;**9**(2):e14746. DOI: 10.2196/14746

[92] Abner M, Wong PK, Cheng JC. Battery lifespan enhancement strategies for edge computing-enabled wireless Bluetooth mesh sensor network for structural health monitoring. Automation in Construction. 2022;**140**:104355. DOI: 10.1016/j.autcon.2022.104355

[93] Kuchenmüller T, Chapman E, Takahashi R, Lester L, Reinap M, Ellen M, et al. A comprehensive monitoring and evaluation framework for evidence to policy networks. Evaluation and Program Planning. 2022;**91**:102053. DOI: 10.1016/j.evalprogplan.2022.102053

[94] O'Connor FK, Chen D, Sharma P, Adsett J, Hwang R, Roberts L, et al. Physiological responses to sit-to-stand and six-minute walk tests in heart failure: A randomised trial. Heart, Lung and Circulation. 2025;**20**:789-797. DOI: 10.1016/j.hlc.2025.03.002

[95] Petersen CB, Eriksen L, Dahl-Petersen IK, Aadahl M, Tolstrup JS. Self-rated physical fitness and measured cardiorespiratory fitness, muscular strength, and body composition. Scandinavian Journal of Medicine & Science in Sports. 2021;**31**(5):1086-1095. DOI: 10.1111/sms.13918

[96] Mathunjwa ML, Djarova-Daniels T, Shaw I, Mugandani S, Shaw BS. Short duration high-intensity interval taekwondo training substantially improves body composition and physical fitness in previously-trained individuals: A proof-of-concept study. Archives of Budo Science of Martial Arts and Extreme Sports. 2020;**16**:221-226

[97] Sornpaisarn B, Limmade Y, Pengpid S, Jayasvasti I, Chhoun P, Somphet V, et al. Assessing data availability of NCD prevention and control in six ASEAN countries based on WHO global monitoring framework and the progress monitor indicators. BMC Public Health. 2023;**23**(1):272. DOI: 10.1186/s12889-023-15165-1

[98] Mason S, Mumford SW. Mixing methods in program evaluation. In: Research Handbook on Program Evaluation. Cheltenham, UK: Edward Elgar Publishing; 2024. pp. 280-303. DOI: 10.4337/9781803928289.00024

[99] Pati S, Mahapatra P, Kanungo S, Uddin A, Sahoo KC. Managing

multimorbidity (multiple chronic diseases) amid COVID-19 pandemic: A community based study from Odisha, India. Frontiers in Public Health. 2021;**8**:584408. DOI: 10.3389/fpubh.2020.584408

[100] Sarmah N, Sibiya MN, Khoza TE. A model for promoting breast self-examination among rural South African women in KwaZulu-Natal. Health SA Gesondheid (Online). 2025;**30**:1-8. DOI: 10.4102/hsag.v30i0.2777

[101] Vannier C, Campbell M, Kingham S. Pathways to urban health and well-being: Measuring and modelling of community services' in a medium size city. Geospatial Health. 2020;**15**(1):156-167. DOI: 10.4081/gh.2020.808

[102] Maziwisa MR, Chigwata TC. The Federal-Local Connection: The South African case. In: Local Governance in Multi-Layered Systems: A Comparative Legal Study in the Federal-Local Connection. Vol. 11. Cham: Springer Nature Switzerland; 2023. pp. 373-399

[103] Nass SJ, Amankwah FK, DeVoe JE, Benjamin GC, National Academies of Sciences, Engineering, and Medicine. Community-centered and community-engaged care. In: Ending Unequal Treatment: Strategies to Achieve Equitable Health Care and Optimal Health for All. Washington, DC: National Academies Press; 2024. p. 23

[104] Tereshchenko E, Salmela E, Melkko E, Phang SK, Happonen A. Emerging best strategies and capabilities for university–industry cooperation: Opportunities for MSMEs and universities to improve collaboration. A literature review 2000-2023. Journal of Innovation and Entrepreneurship. 2024;**13**(1):28. DOI: 10.1186/s13731-024-00386-4

[105] Paul MF. The legal framework and capacity of Uganda police force in eradicating narcotic drugs: A case of Kampala metropolitan policing area [Thesis]

[106] World Health Organization. Global Accelerated Action for the Health of Adolescents (AA-HA!): Guidance to Support Country Implementation. Geneva, Switzerland: World Health Organization; 2023

Chapter 4

Perspective Chapter: The Role of Exercise to Improve the Functional Mobility of the Elderly

Bernelee Denize Doherty and Terry Jeremy Ellapen

Abstract

Aging impacts the elderly physiological and cognitive abilities, leading to a reduced quality of life. Physiologically, they may experience deterioration in muscle strength and endurance, aerobic capacity, decline in sensory functions such as hearing and vision, and susceptibility to chronic diseases like cardiorespiratory disease, cancer and stroke. Cognitively, they can experience memory loss, slower mental processing speed, and challenges with word recall. Some elderly individuals experience osteoporosis, which may predispose them to fractures, limiting their bone strength. Muscles lose their extensibility, potentially predisposing them to arthritis and osteoarthritis. A common muscle condition among the elderly is sarcopenia. Collectively, the loss of muscle strength and endurance, muscle extensibility and proprioception has been cited as contributing influences of poor ability to live independent lives. The sit-to-stand maneuver (STSM) is a reputable motor test to assess an elderly individual's functional capacity. Many elderly individuals struggle with the daily act of STSM. Regular exercise and physical activity maintain muscle strength and endurance, joint flexibility, muscle extensibility, and proprioception. The benefits collectively reduce the risk of neuro-musculoskeletal and hypokinetic diseases. This chapter specifically reviews how exercise improves the elderly ability to STSM.

Keywords: aging, elderly, exercise, sarcopenia, sit-to-stand maneuver

1. Introduction

Over the course of life, an individual's physiological, anatomical and cognitive abilities are characterized into different stages. From birth to 21 years, the muscular, skeletal, nervous, cognitive, cardiovascular and respiratory systems develop in size, strength, and prowess. The age strata of 20 to 40 years marks the peak of an individual's physiological and anatomical functional state, where cognitive ability reaches peak performance during the age strata of 40 to 60 years [1]. The aging process starts as early as in the third decade of life with the most significant changes observed in the fifth decade [1, 2]. Individuals aged 60 years and above are therefore referred to as elderly or senior citizens [1, 2]. The aging process rapidly accelerates among individuals over 65 years. However, the remarkable improvement in geriatric medicine has enabled the elderly population to live longer and it is predicted to double this special population size by the year 2050 reaching approximately 1.5 billion, which will then be approximately 16% of the global population [3]. This increase is largely due to advance medicine and health awareness, but unfortunately the increased life expectancy is also synonymous with increased frailty, characterized by common conditions among the elderly such as sarcopenia, mobility impairments and the onset of chronic non-communicable diseases, which will undoubtedly burden the health care sector, raising many health equity questions [4–6]. The ability of health care workers to determine functional capacity of an individual is of vital importance. The functional reach test, time-up-and go test, hand grip strength and the sit-to-stand maneuver (STSM) are but a few assessment tools mimicking activities frequently performed in daily life [4]. Regular physical activity and clinically evident based exercise programs is demonstrated to improve the elderly person's quality of life thereby delaying or even reversing age-related physiological and cognitive declines [7]. Exercise programs should include aerobic exercises to improve cardiovascular health, endurance and promote healthy weight (body mass) management, strength training to prevent age-related loss of muscle mass (sarcopenia), maintaining functional independence and preventing risks of falling. Joint range of motion exercises is targeted to maintain mobility of the joints and muscle extensibility thereby reducing arthritis and osteoarthritis [1]. Proprioception training improves balance and coordination, thereby increasing sensory function and preventing incidence and/or risk of falls [1].

2. The aging process

Aging is a natural physiological process commonly determined by an individual's "chronological age," which refers to the number of years a person has lived from birth. However, the human body is a complex organism with multiple physiological and anatomical functions, which has led scientists and physiologists to consider the concept of "biological age." Medical scientists and physiologists suggest that biological age is a better concept than chronological age. Biological age estimates the functional state of your body based on molecular and physiological markers, rather than chronological time. While chronological age is fixed, biological age is influenced by lifestyle, environment and genetics, and can predict disease risks and mortality more accurately than your chronological age (birth date). Measures such as DNA methylation and blood biomarkers are used to evaluate biological age, offering insights into one's longevity and potential for interventions to promote a person's longevity [8, 9]. The tendency to lose height with old age is largely due to changes in bones, muscles, joints, intervertebral discs size and individuals typically lose one-half (1 cm) every 10 years after age 40 years [5]. Although very rare maximal life expectancy may reach 120 years and may partially be determined by inherited genes, other factors that impact age include living healthily, physical activity, balanced diet and being emotionally stable [8]. The mean global life expectancy is 73 years.

3. Methodology

This chapter synthesizes the contextual evidence of predisposing factors influencing the geriatric ability to independently perform the STSM. The authors (BDD, TJE) first established the scope (predisposing factors influencing the geriatric ability to independently complete the STSM) and *a priori* propositions (e.g., physiological impact of aging and the biomechanical influences of aging). The authors thereafter completed a focused horizon-scanning to verify terminology, typical exposure ranges and feasibility considerations using popular key references only to triangulate concepts, not to perform an exhaustive review. Evidence were organized into domains (physiology, biomechanics, function and ergonomic options), and points of uncertainty were explicitly identified. This approach afforded clarity of the biomechanical mechanism, clinical physiological plausibility, it does not claim systematic coverage of the literature and avoids the quantitative synthesis by design.

3.1 Physiological impact of aging

Decreased bone density (osteoporosis and osteopenia), muscle mass (sarcopenia) and aerobic capacity along with an increase in adipose tissue are considered normal characteristics of aging [5]. Osteopenia is lower-than-normal bone density, a precursor to osteoporosis, while osteoporosis is a more severe stage where bones are significantly weakened and fragile, making fractures much more likely, with the key difference being the degree of bone loss measured by T-scores (osteopenia: −1 to −2.5; osteoporosis: −2.5 or lower). Sarcopenia is the progressive, age-related loss of skeletal muscle mass, strength and function, leading to weakness, balance issues, falls and difficulty with daily activities, increasing frailty and mortality risk.

The human body is made up of fat, lean mass (muscles and organs) bones and water. Muscle fibers experience depressed capacity to produce proteins, which combat a decrease in muscle cells, fibers and tissue along with the total loss of muscle power, muscle bulk and muscle strength of all major muscle groups, particularly among the deltoids, biceps brachii, triceps brachii, hamstrings, quadriceps femoris and gastrocnemius muscles [5]. Changes are more prominent in fast-twitch muscle fibers as compared to slow-twitch fibers resulting in alarming strength declines among the elderly from 1.5% per year to almost 3% per year over the age of 60 [5]. A decline in muscle mass due to aging is often accompanied with the reduction in muscle strength and endurance among the elderly is termed "sarcopenia" [6]. Sarcopenia has been linked to higher incidences of neuromusculoskeletal injuries associated with falls, fractures and mobility decline thereby reducing one's quality of life and loss of dependency [6]. Sarcopenia poses a greater public health threat especially among women as compared to men. Men generally have greater volume of muscle mass and a shorter life expectancy as compared to women [5].

Hormonal disorders among women also affect the metabolism of bones as well as muscles, and estrogen production, which are considered important for the remodeling of bones and soft tissues, which become compromised with age, leading to chronic bone disorders such as osteoporosis [6, 10]. Osteoporosis is characterized by the decrease in bone density and deteriorated bone microarchitecture. Despite global incidence osteoporosis, this osteological phenomenon often goes underdiagnosed. Empirical investigations have suggested that early diagnosis through bone mineral density (BMD) testing and the implementation of appropriate exercise, and nutritional and pharmacological intervention strategies are essential to prevent fractures and mobility loss in women [10, 11].

As an individual age, their water and/or fluid content within their tissue as well as their cartilage decreases causing muscles to lose extensibility and lengthen, which adds to muscle stiffness and decreased range of motion. As cartilage deteriorates, the bones of the joint begin to grind against one another (crepitus) causing musculoskeletal pain, stiffness and impair movement [5, 12]. Osteoarthritis is a chronic degenerative disease characterized by the breakdown of cartilage in joints and one of the most common forms of arthritis. There are a lot of contributing factors, such as obesity, joint injury and genetic predisposition, but the leading factor contributing to the onset of osteoarthritis is the aging process. Medical scientists and physiologists have predicted that the growing geriatric global population along with increase of obesity and metabolic diseases is expected to double the number of elderly individuals with osteoarthritis by the year 2030, with approximately 50% of cases appearing to be within the geriatric age strata [12].

Age-related kinanthropometry change differs between men and women, with men often gaining body mass until the age of 55 years before starting to lose body mas due to the decline in testosterone levels [5]. Women usually gain body mass until the age of 67–69 years and then begin to lose body mass [5]. These body mass losses later in an individual's life occur because adipose tissue replaces lean muscle mass. Adipose tissue generally aggregates around the center of the body and insulates the organs referred to as central obesity, which has become an alarming health concern among the modern society. Obesity is a complex disease characterized by excessive fat accumulation causing impaired health leading to premature mortality. Obesity is considered as one of the major risk factors causing the onset of non-communicable diseases (NCDs) [5]. Approximately 2.3 billion individuals are overweight with more than 700 million elderly individuals being obese, the elderly onset of obesity contributes to chronic diseases and mobility impairments and a source of much debate on treatment and recommendations.

Obesity is strongly linked to an increased predisposition of cardiovascular diseases (CVD) predominately because it contributes to increasing one's risk of developing hypertension (high blood pressure), diabetes mellitus and elevated cholesterol, as well as morphological (structure) and physiological (functional) changes in the heart. Due to obesity, the heart has to work harder among overweight and/or obese individuals, potentially contributing to heart failure and atrial fibrillation.

Obesity is a cardinal risk for the onset of type 2 diabetes mellitus because excess body fat leads to insulin resistance and impaired insulin secretion, a condition sometimes called "diabesity." Overweight and obese individuals' cells become less responsive to insulin, crucial for regulating blood glucose within the body. These individuals develop a resistance to insulin. Insulin resistance causes the pancreas to produce more insulin to compensate, resulting in the pancreas become damaged and unable to keep up with the increased demand. Aging does not influence how much an individual eats; therefore, it is safe to say decreased energy expenditure among the elderly is a major cause of obesity. Obesity occurs when energy intake exceeds energy expenditure. The possible causes of obesity in the elderly are demonstrated in "**Figure 1**" including several genetic, social and environmental factor [5, 13, 14].

Fractures due to the loss of bone density are common in the vertebral column, hip and wrist, which greatly affect the geriatric individuals' mobility and quality of life [11]. Loss of muscle mass and strength and reduced joint motion with the decrease in bone density are all factors of fall risk among the elderly. One third of geriatric individuals aged 65 years and above experience fall incidences every year, rising to 50% in those aged over 80 years [4, 6, 13]. Although problematic the risk of falls can be detected early, successful exercise intervention programs can be implemented. Clinically based exercise programs may prevent or even reverse the onset of these conditions [4].

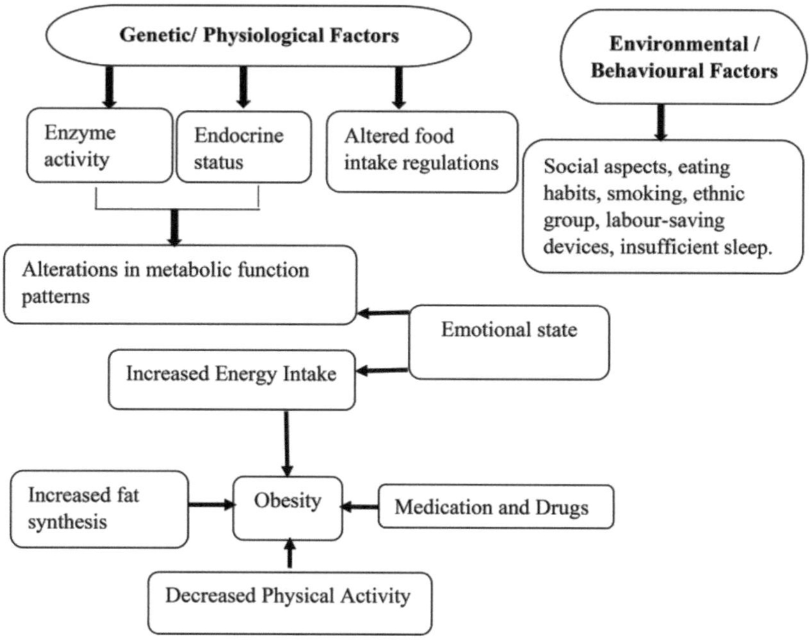

Figure 1.
Causes of obesity.

3.2 Cognitive impact of aging

Elderly individuals start to experience mild cognitive declines starting around 60 years of age, and these age-related changes are the outcome of both distal and proximal life events. Distal life events are those of life experiences including culture, physical and social conditions influencing cognitive functioning and development [5]. Proximal decline includes processing speed, size of working memory, sensory loss and inhibition of extraneous environmental stimuli treating mobility and overall quality of life in the elderly [5]. Brain volume peaks in the early 20s and progressively declines with old age. Individuals may start noticing subtle changes in their ability to remember or focus on more than one task when they reach their 40s, and this is because the cortex of the brain starts to shrink at age 40 years. Blood flow in the brain decreases with age causing the brain to also get less efficient in recruiting patterns and cell-to-cell communication decreasing the ability of the brain to learn. Perceptual motor skills also decline with age. Age-related sensory loss includes hearing loss, taste acuity and vision affecting elderly's ability to read, drive and ultimately their balance putting them at risk of injuries like falls and fractures [5].

Aging brings about the fear of loss in brain function among the elderly, with neurological conditions such as dementia (Alzheimer's disease) and other conditions like Parkinson's disease or sudden stroke (cerebrovascular event) [5]. Alzheimer's and Parkinson's diseases are progressive neurological pathologies commonly observed among the elderly. Alzheimer's disease is the most common type of pre-senile and senile dementia caused by the death of nerve cells and tissue in the brain affecting overall brain functions. Alzheimer's disease is characterized through memory loss, changes in personality and behavior like depression, social withdrawals, mood swings, distrust in others, irritability and aggressiveness [5]. The second leading cause of death globally is strokes (cerebrovascular events) [15]. A stroke occurs when blood flow to the brain is interrupted either due to a blockage (ischemic stroke) or bleeding (hemorrhagic stroke). Stroke treatment and prevention strategies are lacking and not always followed [15]. Stroke exercise rehabilitation programs involves physical activity and exercises to assist individuals to regain lost motor skills, increase their muscle strength and improve their proprioception, which collectively reduce the risk of future cerebrovascular events. Exercise rehabilitation programs should include aerobic exercise (such as walking), range of motion exercises (flexibility), strength training and proprioception. A customized exercise rehabilitation plan is often prescribed and supervised by a physiotherapist, occupational therapist and/or exercise therapist (biokineticist).

4. Functional mobility assessment tools in the elderly

The fundamental skills required to independently care for oneself including eating and bathing and having basic functional mobility are collectively termed activities of daily living (ADL), which serve as an indicator of an individual's functional status [16]. Functional fitness, although traditionally associated with the active young or middle-aged population, has gained popularity for the critical role it plays among the elderly. Strength, flexibility, dynamic balance and aerobic fitness are deemed vital in accomplishing everyday tasks [17]. One major challenge primary caregiver experience is preventing decline in functional mobility among the elderly. The ability to identify premature reduction in functional mobility among the elderly is of paramount importance because physiotherapists, occupational therapists and biokineticists will be able to identify individuals who are not yet functionally disabled, but who are at high risk for functional disability [18, 19]. Assessing these components of fitness may detect weakness and prevent functional decline [17]. Numerous functional screening tests have been proposed to identify and aid the healthcare provider to improve functional mobility among the elderly as well as reducing falls, and these tests include the functional reach test, the timed up and go test and the 30-sec sit-to-stand maneuver [20–22]. These tests are deemed pragmatic as they take into consideration safety, facility, portability and financial cost. The functional reach test (**Figure 2**) requires a participant to stand comfortably next to a wall on which a meter stick will be placed at the acromion level of the preferred limb for reaching. Participants will be asked to reach as far as possible without stepping forward or touching the wall. The distance will be measured on the meter stick using the third finger. This test is one of many balances test used in the elderly as standing balance is considered essential for daily activities [23].

Hand grip strength is associated with a greater risk of frailty and functional decline in the elderly as age-related loss in muscle mass called sarcopenia contributes toward frailty in the elderly. Hand grip dynamometry has therefore been widely used as a diagnostic tool toward frailty in the elderly [24]. The timed up and go test proposed by Podsiadlo and Richardson [24] measured the time to complete a series of movement tasks such as sit-to-stand (STS) and gait for evaluating transferring, sitting and standing abilities among the elderly. The 30-sec STSM test (**Figure 3**) proposed by Jones et al. [25] measures the number of STSM repetitions completed within a 30-second time duration to evaluate the elderly individual's ability to sit-to-stand. Both tests utilize daily living activities as the movement task and employ simple measurement tools such as a tape measure, chair and a stopwatch [25]. The STSM is a transitional movement frequently performed by humans involving the act of repeatedly

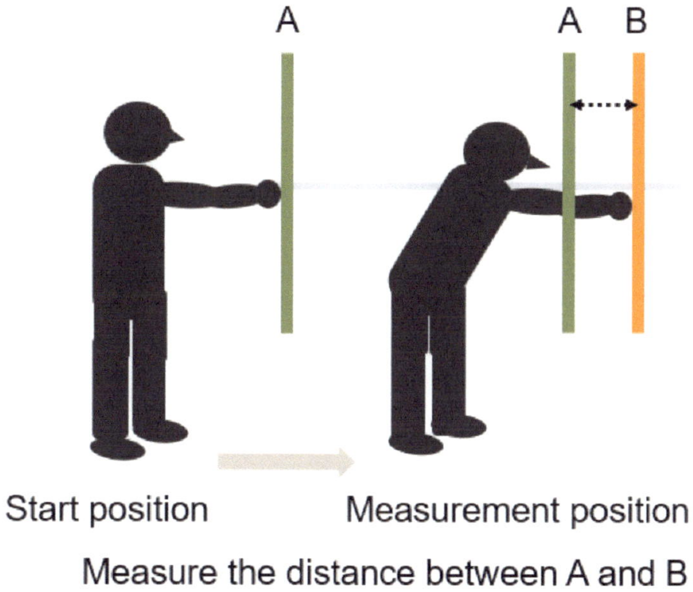

Figure 2.
Functional reach test.

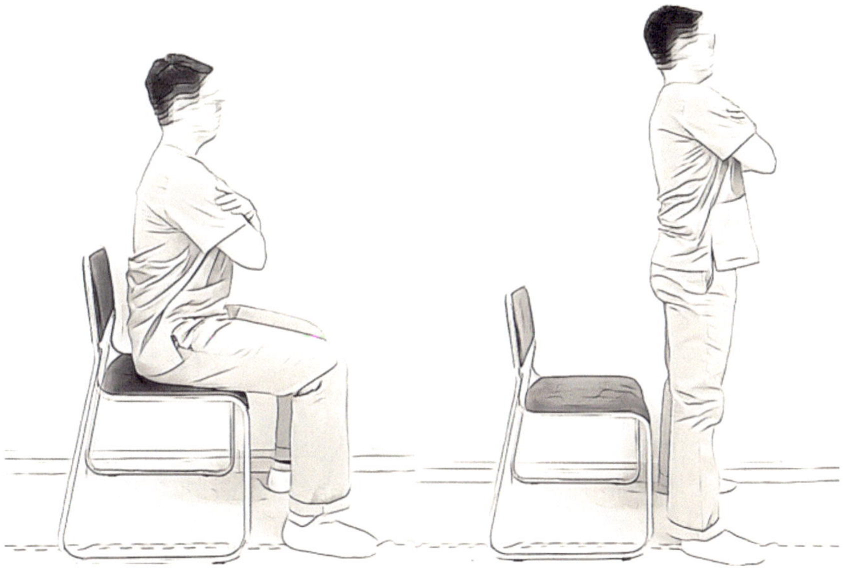

Figure 3.
Sit-to-stand maneuver.

standing up and sitting down from a chair and considered fundamental to most basic activities of daily living [26–28]. Rising from a chair to a standing position is considered a prerequisite for other functional activities such as walking, toileting and dressing. Given the importance of the ability to rise from a chair to a standing position the STSM test has emerged as the most relevant, affordable and potentially effective assessment to identify and improve the functionality mobility among elderly individuals [27].

5. Exercise therapy in the elderly

The benefits of regular physical activity, sport and exercise are widespread with exercise interventions proven to be effective means to improve physiological functioning, decrease risk and onset of chronic diseases such as cardiovascular and metabolic diseases, cancer, depression, arthritis, and osteoporosis reducing fall risk and improving longevity in the elderly [29, 30]. The American College of Sports Medicine advocated that the elderly may also enjoy exercise induce benefits to arrest hypokinetic diseases associated with aging. Exercise programs for the elderly should include gait training, muscle strength and endurance training, flexibility exercises, proprioception, and aerobic exercises (**Table 1**) [29, 30]. The World Health Organization (WHO) recommends that individuals over the age of 65 years should practice aerobic physical activity for at least 150 minutes of moderate in intensity or 75 minutes of high intensity per week. High-intensity exercise generally means increasing one's heart rate to 70 to 95% of their maximum heart rate (MHR). Moreover, elderly people should perform strengthening exercises at least twice a week and balance exercises at least three times a week [30].

Exercise is considered essential for health, especially among the geriatric as it increases muscle mass, reduces body fat and improves muscle strength, endurance, immune functioning and combat cardiovascular diseases. **Table 2** shows an example exercise program to improve the functional mobility of the elderly [32].

Mode	Picture	Intensity
	Warm-up	
Stationary cycling	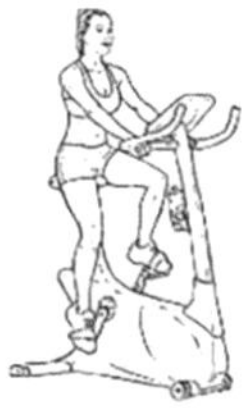	10 min (40% of heart rate reserve)
	Flexibility	
Bicep stretch	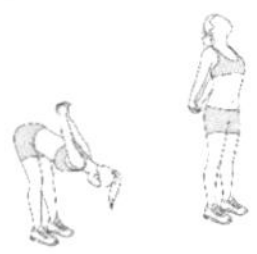	Point of mild discomfort (Hold 15–20 sec)
Triceps stretch	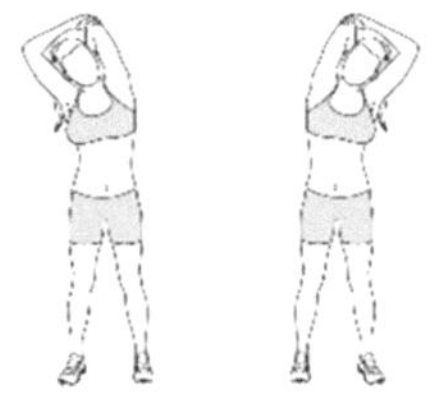	Point of mild discomfort (Hold 15–20 sec)
Doorway stretch	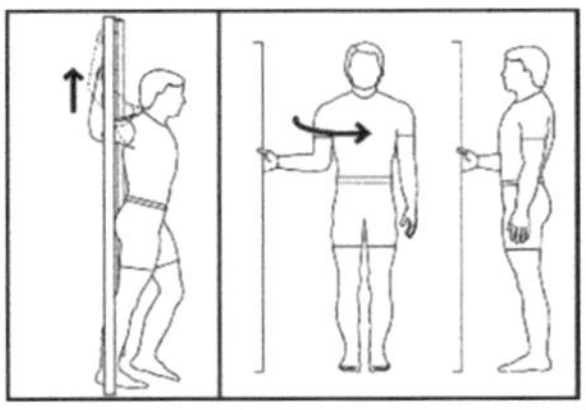	Point of mild discomfort (Hold 15–20 sec)

Mode	Picture	Intensity
Seated H hamstring stretch	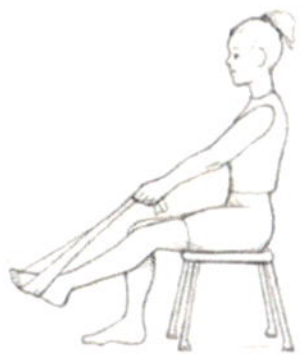	Point of mild discomfort (Hold 15–20 sec)
Quadriceps stretch	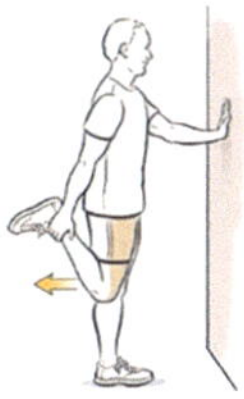	Point of mild discomfort (Hold 15–20 sec)
Standing calf stretch	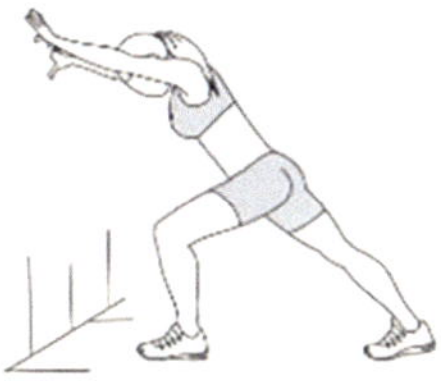	Point of mild discomfort (Hold 15–20 sec)
	Strengthening	
Seated bicep curls	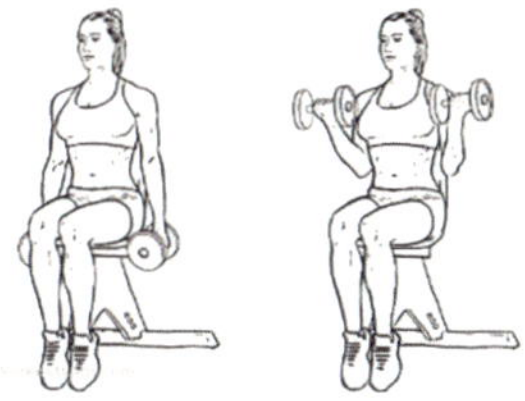	2 Sets, 8–12 Reps
Shoulder external rotation	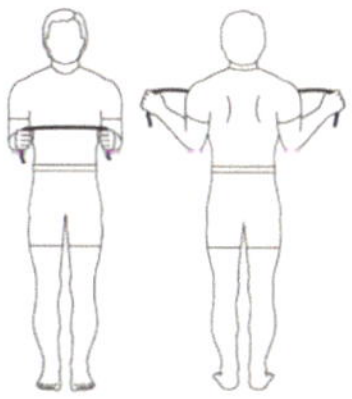	2 Sets, 8–12 Reps
Seated rows	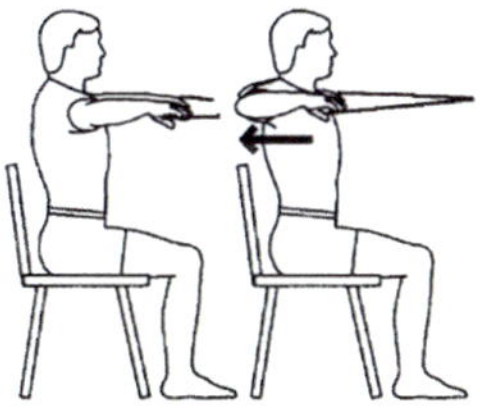	2 Sets, 8–12 Reps
Standing press-ups	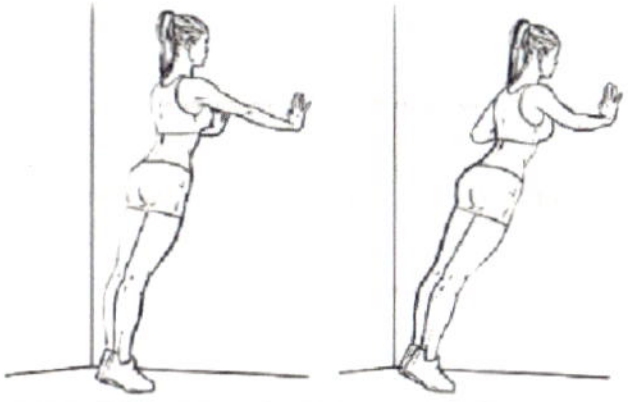	2 Sets, 8–12 Reps

Mode	Picture	Intensity
Seated torso twist	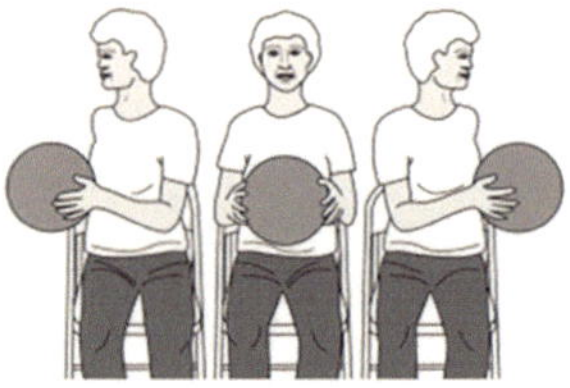	2 Sets, 8–12 Reps
Standing abductions	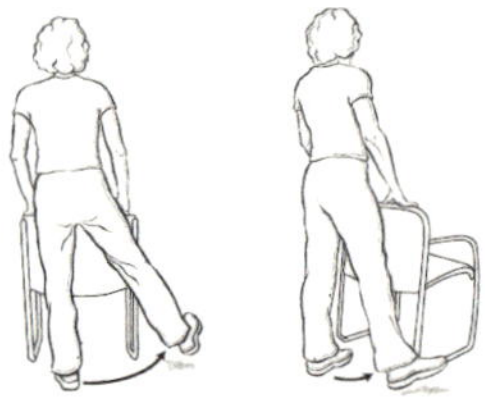	2 Sets, 8–12 Reps
Seated leg extensions	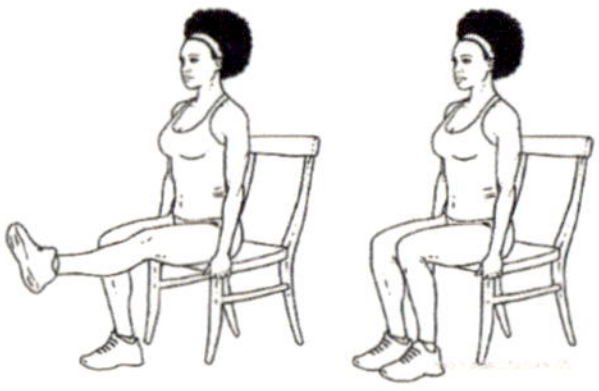	2 Sets, 8–12 Reps
Standing calf raises	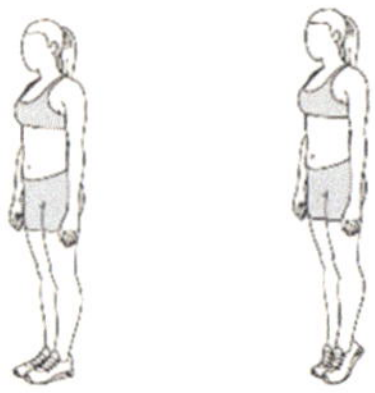	2 Sets, 8–12 Reps
	Proprioception	
Standing one leg (Eyes open/ closed)	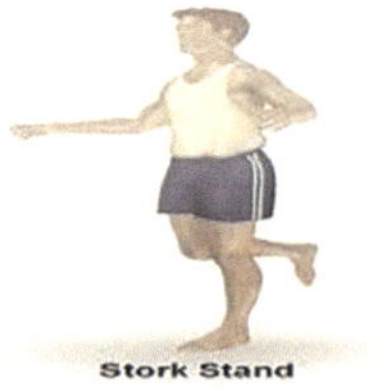	2 Sets, 10 Sec hold
	Cool-down	
Stationary cycling	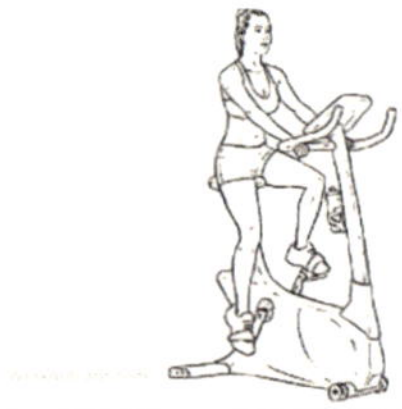	5 min (40% of heart rate reserve)

Table 1.
Example exercises for the elderly.

Component of physical fitness	Frequency	Intensity	Duration	Mode
Cardiorespiratory	>5 days/ wk.	On a scale of 0–10, 5–6 for moderate intensity and 7–8 for vigorous intensity	30–60 min a day of moderate intensity, 20–30 min a day of vigorous intensity	Any exercise that does not pose orthopedic stress. Aquatic exercise, stationary cycle and walking
Resistance	>2 days/ wk.	Light weight (40–50% 1RM), moderate-to-vigorous intensity (60–80% 1RM)	8–10 exercises involving all major muscle groups, 1–3 Sets of 8–12 repetitions each	Progressive weight training, calisthenic and stair climbing
Flexibility	>2 days/ wk.	Stretch to the point of slight discomfort.	Hold stretches for 30–60 seconds	Static stretches for each muscle group

Table 2.
Exercise therapy plan prescribed in the American College of Sports Medicine [31].

5.1 Effects of exercise

5.1.1 Sarcopenia

Exercise should be considered an essential strategy in targeting age-related sarcopenia. Exercise therapy will combat sarcopenia, with the adherence to resistance training, which will increase muscle strength and endurance, physical function and hypertrophy. Aerobic exercise causes increased ATP production within mitochondria of skeletal muscles, reducing the expressions of catabolic genes and increasing protein synthesis. Resistance exercise increases the size and cross-sectional areas of muscle fibers (hypertrophy), especially fast-twitch muscle fibers along with increased protein synthesis and muscle fiber hypertrophy promote greater muscle force generating ability [32]. Different types of pf exercises will recruit the different muscle fibers, as well change the undifferentiated satellite muscle fibers into either type 1 or type 2 muscle fibers. These benefits will reverse the sarcopenia and improve the elderly individual's quality of life.

5.1.2 Osteoporosis

Low bone density is an important risk factor for fractures among the elderly and therefore a key aspect to address for the prevention of osteoporosis. Reduced activity with old age causes unloading of the skeletal system resulting in decreased bone density, and exercise is known for stimulating bone growth preserving bone density and preventing fall risk in the elderly [10, 33]. Habitual strength training increases bone density by imposing stress onto the bones, which stimulates bone cells to become stronger and more resilient. This process, known as osteogenic loading, leads to stronger, denser bones, limiting the risk of osteopenia, osteoporosis and fractures. In order to achieve optimal benefits, resistance training should be performed at a moderate intensity, with consistency and a focus on symmetric development of all muscle groups and the appendicular and axial skeleton.

5.1.3 Arthritis

Exercise relieves pathological changes associated with osteoarthritis by decreasing pain, enhancing muscle strength and improving joint stiffness. Many exercises have therapeutic effects on osteoarthritis, and low aerobic exercises are mostly used as it reduces pain, prevents cartilage degradation and improves body function [12]. Regular exercise and physical activity increase the secretion of synovial fluid, which increases joint lubrication thereby reducing crepitus [34]. Stronger muscles surrounding joints provide better support, stability and joint congruency, which reduce the stress placed on the joint cartilage. Regular exercise and physical activity increases blood flow to the cartilage of arthritic joints, thereby delivering the nutrients needs to replenish lubrication within the joint.

5.1.4 Obesity

As obesity is an excessive fat accumulation in adipose tissue, reducing adipose tissue is considered one way of reducing excess body mass within an individual, thereby combating obesity. Two effective methods exist that are dietary modifications and energy expenditure modifications (regular exercise and physical activity). Therefore, exercise is seen as an effective method in combating obesity among the elderly [33, 34]. Expending calories through physical activity, combined with a calories reduced nutritional plan, creates a calorie deficit that results in weight loss. Body fat and body mass loss occurs from decreasing calories. However, the only way to maintain weight loss is to engage in regular exercise, physical activity and sport. Regular exercise and physical activity increase one's resting metabolic rate, which translates as the body's ability to expend more calories when at rest. Habitual exercise, sports and physical activity decrease obesity by activating beta-adrenergic signaling, which facilitates the lipolysis of stored fat (triacylglycerols) in adipose tissue, thereby discharging free fatty acids to be used as energy (fuel) by working (active) muscles. This process, called beta lipidization, which additional increases blood flow to adipose tissue and muscles, facilitates fatty acid transport and use. Further, exercise promotes mitochondrial function, enhances fatty acid oxidation in muscle and fat cells and increases the release of beneficial adipokines, ultimately reducing fat mass, improving insulin sensitivity and mitigating inflammation associated with obesity.

5.1.5 Diabetes mellitus

The inability of the body to control blood glucose levels is termed diabetes "to pass through" in Greek and mellitus "sweet" in Latin. Diabetes mellitus can be classified into type 1, type 2, maturity-onset diabetes of the young, gestational diabetes, neonatal diabetes and steroid-induced diabetes. Type 1 and type 2 diabetes are the most common form; however, type 2 diabetes is commonly developed from obesity and old age. Exercise promotes blood glucose absorption as active contraction of muscles increases translocation of type 4 glucose transporters from the cytoplasm of strained muscles [35, 36].

5.1.6 Cardiovascular disease

Aging greatly influences heart and blood vessel health leading to a variety of cardiovascular diseases. Hypertension is one such commonly observed predisposing risk factor in the elderly. It is widely known that exercise decreases systolic blood pressure with about 5 mmHg and diastolic blood pressure with about 3.5 mmHg ultimately reducing the risk of strokes as well as acute coronary disease. Cardiovascular diseases start from a young age; therefore, risk management strategies should start early in order to prevent cardiovascular diseases in the elderly [36, 37].

6. Conclusions

Functional mobility is of paramount importance to maintain independence among the elderly. Physiological and anatomical changes occur with an increase in age bringing about addition challenges. Decline in functional mobility may present itself gradually over many years or occur overnight due to sudden injury incidences. Evidence has confirmed exercise therapy to delay age-related functional decline among the elderly. Exercise interventions may include clinical based or home-based programs and should be cost-effective, entrusting and easily maintained. Special attention should be given to preventative exercise interventions trying to minimize the risks factors for functional decline including obesity, falls and physical inactivity. Exercise interventions should target all age groups to minimize future risk of functional mobility decline. By doing so young people may slow down the aging process by being active, learning new mobility skills and through good treatment of diseases. Exercise plays a vital role in the functional mobility of the elderly and specific and supportive environments have become increasingly important. To minimize the age-related functional decline in the elderly an emphasis should be placed on the importance of exercise to maintain independence, clinical as well as community-based functional fitness tests will have to be performed to identify areas of particular concern and individualized exercise programs will have to be developed, implemented and maintained. Only by doing so can we improve the functional mobility in the elderly population, reducing the burden on the health care sector.

Acknowledgements

The images displaying the exercises were taken from the internet.

Conflict of interest

The authors declare no conflict of interest.

Author details

Bernelee Denize Doherty* and Terry Jeremy Ellapen
Tshwane University of Technology, Pretoria, Gauteng, South Africa

*Address all correspondence to: bddoherty95@gmail.com

References

[1] Ellapen TJ, Ntjana BM, Ribeiro-Wagner C, Paul Y. The role of exercise therapy in the management of Parkinsons disease. In: Neurological Problems in the Elderly-Bridging Current State and New Outlooks. No. 7. United Kingdom: IntechOpen; 2024. DOI: 10.5772/intechopen.1006114

[2] Smith SHL, Reilly P, Bull AMJ. A musculoskeletal modelling approach to explain sit-to-stand difficulties in older people due to changes in muscle recruitment and movement strategies. Journal of Biomechanics. 2020;**98**: 109451

[3] Padeiro M, Santana P, Grant M. Global aging and health determinants in a changing world. In: Aging. Portugal: Academic Press; 2023. pp. 3-30. DOI: 10.1016/B978-0-12-823761-8.00021-5

[4] Shukla B, Bassement J, Vijay V, Yadav S, Hewson D. Instrumented analysis of the sit-to-stand movement for geriatric screening: A systematic review. Bioengineering. 2020;7:1-13

[5] Amarya S, Singh K, Sabharrwal M. Ageing process and physiological changes. In: Gerontology. London, UK: IntechOpen; 2018. pp. 4-24

[6] Su YC, Chang SF, Tsai HC. The relationship between sarcopenia and injury events: A systematic review and meta-analysis of 98,754 older adults. Journal of Clinical Medicine. 2022;**11** (21):6474

[7] Murao Y, Ishikawa J, Tamura Y, Kobayashi F, Toba A, Harada K, et al. Association between physical performance during sit-to-stand motion and frailty in older adults with cardiometabolic diseases: A cross-sectional, longitudinal study. BMC Geriatrics. 2023;**23**(337):1-10. DOI: 10.1186/s12877-023-04011-z

[8] Preston J, Biddell B. The physiology of ageing and how these changes affect older people. Medicine. 2021;**49** (1):1-5

[9] Cologne. General Methods [Internet]. Germany: Institute for Quality and Efficiency in Health Care; 2020. Available from: https://www.ncbi.nlm.nih.gov/books/NBK563107

[10] Pinheiro MB, Oliveira J, Bauman A, Fairhall N, Kwok W, Sherrington C. Evidence on physical activity and osteoporosis prevention for people aged 65+ years: A systematic review to inform the WHO guidelines on physical activity and sedentary behaviour. International Journal of Behavioural Nutrition and Physical Activity. 2020;**17**:150

[11] Keen MU, Barrnett MJ, Anastasopoulou C. Osteoporosis in Females. Treasure Island Florida: Statpearls Publishing; 2025. [Internet]. Available from: https://www.ncbi.nlm.nih.gov/books/NBK559156

[12] Kong H, Wang XQ, Zhang XA. Exercise for osteoarthritis: A literature review of pathology and mechanism. Frontiers in Aging Neuroscience. 2022; **14**:1-20

[13] McKee AM, Morley JE. Obesity in the Elderly. Oregon USA: EndoText.org [Internet]; 2021. Available from: https://www.ncbi.nlm.nih.gov/sites/books/NBK532533

[14] Malenfant J, Batasis JA. Obesity in the geriatric population – A global health perspective. Journal of Global Health Reports. 2019;**3**:e2019045

[15] Sharrief A, Grotta JC. Stroke in the elderly. Geriatric Neurology. 2019;**167**: 394-418

[16] Edemeong PF, Bomgaars L, Sukumaran S, Levy SB. Activities of Daily Living. Treasure Island, Florida: StatPearls Publishing; 2020. Available from: https://digitalcollections.dordt.edu/faculty_work/1222?utm_source=digitalcollections.dordt.edu%2Ffaculty_work%2F1222&utm_medium=PDF&utm_campaign=PDFCoverPages

[17] Cossio-Bolaños M, Vidal-Espinoza R, Villar-Cifuentes I, Correia de Campos LFC, Ramos de Lázari MS, Urra-Albornoz C, et al. Functional fitness benchmark values for older adults: A systematic review. Frontiers in Public Health. 2024;**21**(12):1-12

[18] Hildebrand C, Taylor M, Bradway C. Elder self-neglect: The failure of coping because of cognitive and functional impairments. Journal of the American Association of Nurse Practitioners. 2014;**26**(8):452-462

[19] Roedi KJ, Wilson LS, Fine J. A systematic review and comparison of functional assessments of community-dwelling elderly patients. Journal of the American Association of Nurse Practitioners. 2016;**28**:160-169

[20] Duncan PW, Weiner DK, Chandler J, Studenski S. Functional reach: A new clinical measure of balance. Journal of Gerontology. 1990;**45**(6):192-197

[21] Bohannon RW. Comfortable and maximum walking speed of adults aged 20-79 years: Reference values and determinants. Age and Ageing. 1997;**26**(1):15-19

[22] Podsiadlo D, Richardson S. The timed "Up & Go": A test of basic functional mobility for frail elderly persons. Journal of the American Geriatrics Society. 1991;**39**(2):142-148

[23] Bohannon RB, Wolfson LI, White WB. Functional reach of older adults: Normative reference values based on new and published data. Physiotherapy. 2017;**103**(4):387-391

[24] Benton MJ, Spicher JM, Silva-Smith AL. Validity and reliability of handgrip dynamometry in older adults: A comparison of two widely used dynamometers. PLoS One. 2022;**17**(6):1-15

[25] Jones CJ, Rikli RE, Beam WC. A 30-s chair-stand test as a measure of lower body strength in community-residing older adults. Research Quarterly for Exercise and Sport. 1999;**70**(2):113-119

[26] Slaughter SE, Wagg AS, Jones CA, Schopflocher D, Ickert C, Bampton E, et al. Mobility of vulnerable elders study: Effect of the sit-to-stand activity on mobility, function, and quality of life. Journal of the Post-Acute and Long Term Care Medical Association. 2015;**16**(2): 138-143

[27] Wisnesky UD, Olson J, Paul P, Dahlke S, Slaughter SE, Lopes V. Sit-to-stand activity to improve mobility in older people: A scoping review. International Journal of Old People Nursing. 2020;**15**:1-11

[28] De Koning C, Miller M, Tucker C, Ellapen TJ. An anteriorly tilted pelvis adversely influence the elderly's ability to sit to stand? African Journal for Physical, Health Education, Recreation and Dance. 2014;**20**(2:2):646-654

[29] Kwak CJ, Kim YL, Lee SM. Effects of elastic-band resistance exercise on balance, mobility and gait function, flexibility and fall efficacy in elderly people. Journal of Physical Therapy Science. 2016;**28**(11):3189-2016

[30] Hasselman V, Oesch P, Fernandez-Luque L, Bachmann S. Are exergames promoting mobility an attractive alternative to conventional self-regulated exercises for elderly people in a rehabilitation setting? Study protocol of a randomized controlled trial. BMC Geriatrics. 2015;**15**:108

[31] Kluwer W. ACSM'S Guidelines for Exercise Testing and Prescription. 11th ed. Philadelphia: American Collage of Sports Medicine; 2018

[32] Yoo SZ, No MH, Heo JW, Park DH, Kang JH, Kim SH, et al. Role of exercise in age-related sarcopenia. Journal of Exercise Rehabilitation. 2018;**14**(4): 551-558

[33] Niemiro GM, Rewane A, Algotar AM. Exercise and Fitness Effect on Obesity. Treasure Island, Florida: Statpearls Publishing; 2023. [Internet]. Available from: https://www.ncbi.nlm.nih.gov/books/NBK539893/

[34] Ellapen TJ, Swanepoel M, Strydom GL. A comparative review of the rehabilitative professions assisting patients with lower back pain in South Africa. South African Journal of Research in Sport Physical Education Recreation. 2017;**39**(3):1-14. Available from: https://hdl.handle.net/10520/EJC-c378942be

[35] Ciumărnean L, Milaciu MV, Negrean V, Orăsan OH, Vesa SC, Sălăgean O, et al. Cardiovascular risk factors and physical activity for the prevention of cardiovascular diseases. International Journal of Environmental Research and Public Health. 2022;**19**(207):1-16

[36] Sapra A, Bhandari P. Diabetes. Treasure Island, Florida: StatPearls Publishing; 2023 [Internet]. Available from: https://www.ncbi.nlm.nih.gov/books/NBK551501/#:~:text=Diabetes%20mellitus%20(DM)%20is%20a%20metabolic%20disease%2C%20involving%20inappropriately

[37] Lettino M, Mascherbauer J, Nordaby M, Ziegler A, Collet JP, Derumeaux G, et al. Cardiovascular disease in the elderly: Proceedings of the European Society of Cardiology-Cardiovascular Round Table. European Journal of Preventive Cardiology. 2022;**29**(10):1412-1424

Chapter 5

Perspective Chapter: "Move-to-the-Beat, Take the Lead" – The Impact of Active Lifestyle on Neurocognitive Functions

Meha Fatima Aftab

Abstract

Recall that dance that made you feel so energetic despite utilizing your glucose reserves! Did you wonder why you were not tired instead? Exercise has this "not-so-spurious" effect on our brain function and can be beneficial in reducing the rising burden of mental disorders. This chapter aims to highlight the cellular and neurocognitive influences of exercise. Moderate- to-high-intensity exercise increases BDNF and NGF levels, which redirects the brain metabolism to favor the production of excitatory molecules like glutamate and reduced norepinephrine in the fear center, ultimately activating the circuitry involved in the higher cognitive functions. Glutamate and dopamine levels in the cognitive circuitry can increase brain function including learning and memory, thereby reducing risk of neurodegeneration. Contrary to moderate-intensity exercises, high-intensity short-term exercises instead lead to exhaustion and offer lesser benefits. Moderate-intensity training also improves cognitive outcomes by activating language centers, improving word recall and alleviating symptoms in dyslexia and social anxiety while enhancing emotional intelligence scores. Exercise influences interoception by modulating heart rate variability and heart beat evoked potentials (HEPs) in the brain. HEPs reflect a state of interoceptive and emotional processing, necessary to navigate through decision-making. A demonstrated role of exercise also exists in the prevention of cognitive decline in aging. Exercise uncovers the mystery behind the concept of "body-mind" in biopsychosocial model, hence establishing the importance of exercise in improving cognitive outcomes. Moderate-intensity exercises thus hold potential as a therapeutic modality in the rehabilitative treatment of various neurocognitive disorders.

Keywords: exercise, cognition, executive function, memory, interoception, emotion

1. Introduction

The rise in mental disorders calls out for the development of novel therapeutic strategies with minimal side effects and positive global effects in the body. The persistence of these mental disorders can impair cognitive abilities in a person. Cognition is evident in the brain functions including perception, learning and memory, decision-making, language, social cognition, sensation, executive function, and interoception [1]. Conventional pharmacological treatments of mental disorders pose serious adverse effects and cause dependence. Exercise holds critical value in treating metabolic disorders. The behavioral symptoms of mental disorders can be partly explained by the disrupted brain metabolism. Hence, exercise can improve behavioral symptoms by modulating brain metabolism. This chapter highlights important molecular and electrophysiological modulations in response to active lifestyle including evidences from leisure activities and structured exercise paradigms and simultaneously discuss their effects on cognitive and emotional outcomes.

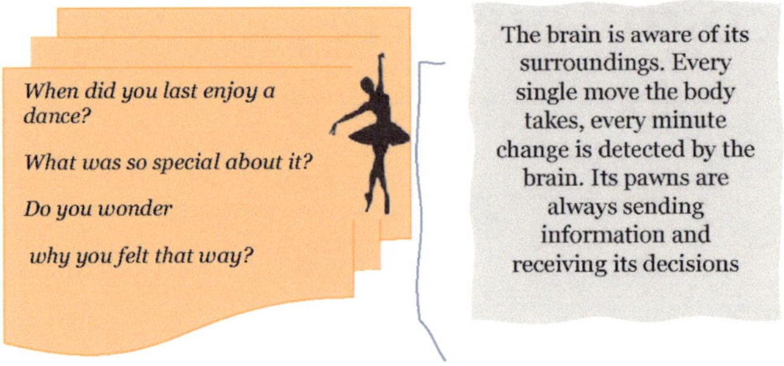

An active lifestyle can significantly influence positive cognitive outcomes. Physical activity can enhance metabolism *via* either non-exercise activity thermogenesis (NEAT), including leisure or daily activities [2], or structured exercise paradigms like strength training [3], aerobic [3], running, pushups, flexibility exercises, walking, circuit training, cardio [3], high-intensity interval training, and moderate-intensity exercises among many others. A well-known mechanism of the effect of exercise is increased blood flow to the regions of blood supply [4]. Brain in this case receives approximately 25–30% of the blood supply [5, 6], hence the observed effects of exercise on brain function. Clinical and public health studies have shown the impressive effects of different types of exercises on cognitive functions.

In this chapter, a detailed discussion on both the effects of non-exercise physical activity and exercise has been placed, while the molecular and electrophysiological effects of exercise are also highlighted in the subsequent section. The studies exploring the influence of non-exercise physical activity are termed as "physical activity," while structured exercise paradigms are discussed as "exercise." **Table 1** summarizes the studies addressing non-exercise physical activity and different exercise paradigms with their health outcomes.

2. Perception

Perception requires reception, organization, and integration of sensory inputs from all over the body. The major types of sensations include hearing, touch, taste, sight, and smell. However, in addition to these well-known sensations the sense of proprioception and interoception are less discussed. We will now look deeper into how exercise impacts each of these senses.

2.1 Sense of sight

Let us start with a very basic notion of "exercise increase blood flow." Having said that, it's not just the peripheral effects. Running, for instance, has shown a direct effect on visual responses by activating narrow-spiking cells [38] that are inhibitory in nature.

Authors	Type of physical activity	Intensity	Duration (minutes)	Study design	Cognitive and/or emotional outcomes
Hu *et al.* [7]	Physical activity in middle school students	Not specified	Not specified (survey)	Cross-sectional, human	Reduced negative emotions, improved social competence and relationships
Neeper *et al.* [8]	Voluntary wheel running (rats)	Not specified	Variable, overnights (2, 4, or 7 days)	Experimental animal (rats)	↑ BDNF mRNA (hippocampus & cortex); ↑ NGF mRNA (hippocampus & cortex)
Liu *et al.* [9]	Ergometer bicycling with adjustable load	60% of Max. HR	20 minutes prior to learning	Experimental, human	Improved second-language learning
Maddock *et al.* [10]	Graded/vigorous aerobic exercise in humans	~85% of age-predicted maximum HR (vigorous)	Not explicitly given, likely several minutes of graded exercise to target HR	Experimental, human, acute	↑ brain lactate (~19%); ↑ Gln (~18%) in visual cortex
Marchant *et al.* [11]	Cycling post-learning	20 min	Moderate vs. high	Experimental	Memory retention modulated by intensity/timing
Jentsch and Wolf [12]	Running	10% treadmill inclination, 0.5, 0.5 m/s every 30 seconds, 85% HRR	~ 20 minutes (until HRR was achieved)	Experimental, human, acute	Promotes consolidation of emotional memory
Li *et al.* [13]	Comparison of low vs. high exercise adolescent groups	Undefined (Same across groups)	LE: 30 min/once a day HE: 30 min/twice a day CON: No exercise	Experimental, human, adolescent	Dose-dependent improvement in inhibitory control
Zimmermann and Chakravarti [14]	Leisure physical Activity	Undefined	Not specified	Human behavioral	Influences decision-making in unrelated domains (altered/improved decision-making performance)
Fonseca *et al.* [15]	Physical exercise affecting nasal volume	Maximum effort test with 25 Watts load	Not specified	Human experimental	Increased nasal volume (improved nasal patency)
Namiranian *et al.* [16]	Moderate-intensity physical activity (varied frequency)	Moderate intensity (stated)	Not specified (based on survey/cross-sectional)	Human observational, cross-sectional	Better olfactory function linked to higher frequency and moderate intensity
Amaya *et al.* [17]	Aerobic exercise in university students	50% HRR Moderate-intensity stepping exercises	30 minutes/day 3 times/week	Non-randomized controlled trial	Improved interoception and cognitive function

Authors	Type of physical activity	Intensity	Duration (minutes)	Study design	Cognitive and/or emotional outcomes
Watson *et al.* [18]	Physical activity in children	50% HRR Bench-step exercise	30 minutes/day 3 times/week	Observational or cross-sectional	Higher activity associated with better inhibitory control in children
Santos *et al.* [19]	Physical activity patterns in adolescents	Not specified	Not specified (observational)	Observational, cross-sectional	Associations between taste sensitivity, food preferences, activity, and nutritional status
Cheng *et al.* [20]	Long-term physical exercise	Moderate or high intensity	30 minutes/day 3 times/week	Quasi-experimental, human	Improved persistent and inhibitory self-control
Gauthier *et al.* [21, 22]	Various physical exercises (systematic review)	Various intensities	Various durations	Systematic review	Effects on taste perception across modalities (improvements or changes)
Marques *et al.* [23]	Physical activity across adulthood (systematic review)	Not specified	Not specified	Systematic review	Bidirectional association between physical activity and dopamine across adulthood
Li *et al.* [24]	Physical activity in children and adolescents	Not specified (various)	Not specified	Systematic review and meta-analysis	Enhanced positive emotions (heightened positive affect)
Wallman-Jones *et al.* [25]	Physical activity (theoretical considerations)	Theoretical, various	Theoretical	Theoretical review	Conceptual insights: PA's potential effects on interoceptive processing and related benefits
Harnish *et al.* [26]	Aerobic exercise + aphasia therapy	45 min/session, 3×/week, 8 weeks	Moderate	RCT	Improved language function in post-stroke aphasia
Coleman *et al.* [27]	Cycling	20 min	Moderate (~65% HRmax)	Within-subject	Faster selective—attention responses
Bullock *et al.* [28]	Cycling	30 min	Moderate	Within-subject	Improved visual selective attention
Ligieza *et al.* [29]	Cycling	30 min	~70% HRmax	Within-subject	Enhanced neural allocation for attention
Swiatkiewicz *et al.* [30]	Treadmill running (rats)	60–90 min to exhaustion	Endurance (24 m/min)	Experimental	↑ Brain Glu/Gln levels (^{1}H-MRS)

DOI: http://dx.doi.org/10.5772/intechopen.1013187

Authors	Type of physical activity	Intensity	Duration (minutes)	Study design	Cognitive and/or emotional outcomes
Erickson *et al.* [31]	Walking	40 min, 3×/week, 12 months	40–60% HRR	RCT	↑ Hippocampal volume (~2%), improved memory
Farzi *et al.* [32]	Treadmill running and resistance ladder (rats)	8 weeks, 4 days/week	Progressive load	Experimental	Improved recognition memory, ↓ AChE
Loprinzi *et al.* [33]	Acute aerobic exercise	15 min	Moderate	Experimental	Improved episodic memory consolidation
Chaire *et al.* [34]	Cycling	20 min	Moderate vs. high	Experimental	Intensity-dependent effects on attention
Pesce *et al.* [35]	Physical education (circuit vs. games)	~40 min	~140 bpm	RCT	Improved free-recall memory
Kimura *et al.* [36]	Dual-task cycling	15 min	Low vs. moderate	Experimental	Different prefrontal cortex activation (fNIRS)
Won *et al.* [37]	Aerobic exercise	Single bout	Moderate	Experimental	↑ Semantic memory activation in older adults

↑: increased; BDNF: brain-derived neurotrophic factor; NGF: nerve growth factor, mRNA: messenger RNA; Gln: glutamine; HR: heart rate; HRR: heart rate reserve; LE: low-intensity exercise; HE: high-intensity exercise; CON: control group; AChE: acetylcholine estrase; ^{1}H-MRS: proton magnetic resonance spectroscopy; fNIRs: functional near-infrared spectroscopy.

Table 1.
A summary of research highlighting the effect of non-exercise physical activity and exercise on health outcomes.

If we dig deeper, running facilitates recovery of amblyopic eye through increased synaptic transmission of vasoactive-intestinal peptide (VIP) [39] in rodent models. Physical activity also influences the molecular changes that are increased expression of brain-derived neurotrophic factor (BDNF) and nerve growth factor (NGF) [8]. Even graded activity *via* bicycle ergometer enhanced glutamate levels in the V1 area of the visual cortex [10], explained by an increase in the brain lactate due to increased oxygen demand during physical activity, which redirects the brain toward amino acid metabolism [40], resulting in release of neurotransmitter levels. The release of excitatory neurotransmitters in the visual cortex thus enhances the visual perception.

Visual perception involves both central and peripheral vision. Distinct areas of visual cortex are responsible for visual clue processing. Excitatory neurotransmission in response to both physical activity and exercise can improve central and peripheral vision. Additionally, sympathetic responses from autonomic nervous system can improve focus. Hence, exercise can act to improve vision *via* central, peripheral, and autonomic pathways.

2.2 Sense of hearing

Hearing is critical for communication. Impaired hearing occurring in sensorineural hearing loss can cause neurodegeneration [41]. Exercise improves hearing by modulating the auditory thresholds. Two months of continuous cycling improves pure tone hearing at 2–4 KHz [42]. Consequently, physical activity measures taken during midlife reduce chances of hearing loss and even improves hearing threshold and word distinction in noise [43]. Similarly three-month aerobic training or stretching added as an adjunct to aphasia therapy exerted the enhanced effects as compared to aphasia therapy alone, resulting in increase in circulating BDNF levels [26]. Some confounding studies show that 50% of maximum work capacity cycling on ergometer for 10 minutes depresses stapedius reflex activity in cochlea resulting in modulation of temporary threshold shift (TTS) in the presence of noise [44]. This temporary threshold shift may serve a protective effect by redirecting attention to the external noise (threats). However, decreased stapedius reflex outputs were observed with high-intensity levels in this case, postulated to be influenced by stapedius muscle contraction and biochemical modifications acting centrally. This confound can be explained by the activation of sympathetic system during exercise, which may dampen the blood flow to stapedius and redirect it to major muscles of the body. Nevertheless, this effect is observed by a 10-minute ergometer cycling and may have differential effects in the long term, a hypothesis that needs further exploration.

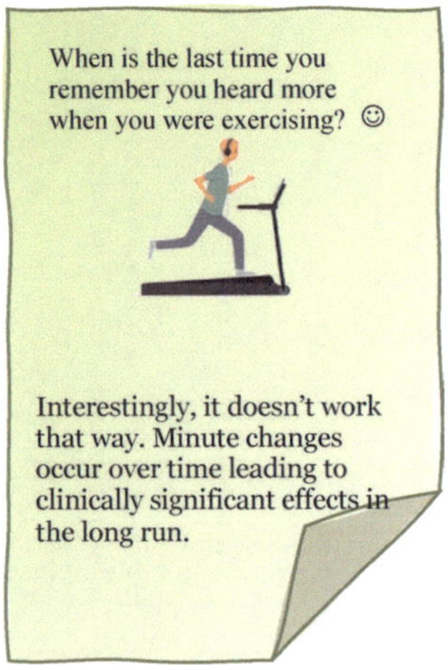

Hearing loss poses serious risk By decreasing perception of environmental auditory cues during movement and social isolation, and limits attention during simultaneous tasks [45]. Hearing loss in older adults is associated with gait speed [46] and poor physical functioning [47], which signifies that while we may not be observing immediate clinical effects of exercise on hearing, long-term impact of poor physical activity may dictate the emergence of hearing impairment. The mechanism of these long-term consequences can be identified by delineating the short-term effects of exercise on hearing.

2.3 Sense of olfaction

Olfaction consists of three main components, odor detection threshold, odor identification, and odor intensity [48]. Odor detection depends on odor concentration in the environment. The loss of olfactory acuity is evident in degenerative and metabolic diseases [49–51], ultimately also impacting the energy intake. Numerous studies have documented the positive impact of exercise, specially aerobic exercise in improving olfaction [52–55].

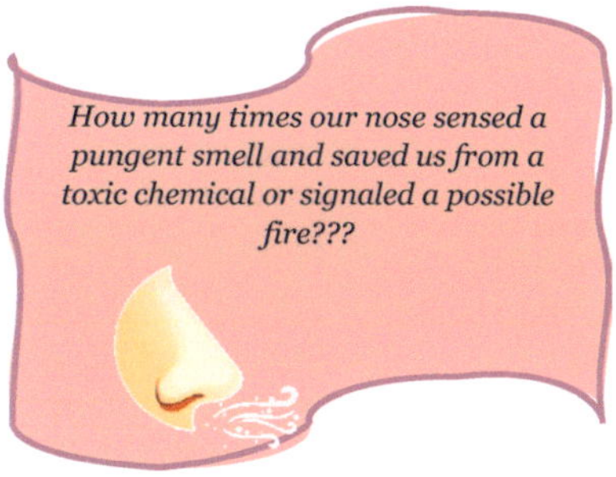

Physical activity can exert the effects on olfaction *via* two possible mechanisms: (1) increasing blood flow to nasal cavity thereby sensitizing the olfactory receptors and (2) enhancing cerebral blood flow, thereby activating brain function. Transient increases in nasal permeability have been reported immediately following aerobic exercise [15], which could be attributed to increased blood flow during the exercise. Contrasting evidences also exist where high-intensity exercise has been linked to exercise induced bronchoconstriction [56] and increased chances of upper tract respiratory infections (URTIs) [57]. Interestingly, the chances of URTIs increase in an open-window time frame spanning from 1 to 9 hours after heavy training [57]; however, moderate-intensity regular exercise has shown protective effects [58], hypothesized to be related to a shift in serum innate immunity proteins [59]. Moderate physical activity improves odds of accurate identification of odors, thereby also enhancing signals for dangerous stimuli like smoke, serving a positive protective effect [16]. The odorant signals are transduced *via* Odorant receptor 83B (OR83B) which works with GPCR signaling. Decreased functioning of OR83B occurs during endurance exercise resulting in resistance to cardiac stress [60], thereby influencing lifespan. While exercise has shown contrasting effects on URT, these are evident mainly with heavy training. Heavy trainings increase oxygen demands thereby enhancing breathing rate, leading to friction in the airway, making it prone to develop infections. Long-term moderate-intensity exercise is rather protective due to improvement in immune function [61].

2.4 Gustation

The contemporary world has seen a rise in metabolic disorders, a result of consumption of high fat/high processed food. This high consumption occurs just to satisfy this one sense out of five!

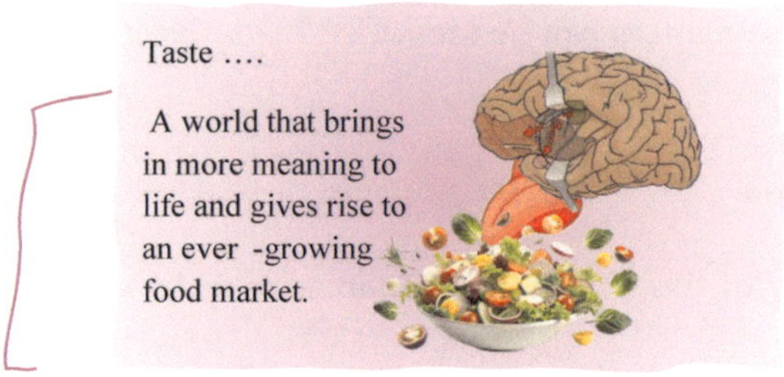

Let us imagine the impact of the sense of taste and get inspired by how we can modulate this picky and pampered sense in our bodies...

Gustation comprises of five distinct tastes: salty, bitter, sweet, sour, and umami. Taste discrimination is tightly linked to food preferences and ultimately nutrition. Taste perception is affected in neurodegenerative disorders [62], leading to malnutrition [63, 64]. Also, we must acknowledge that gustation is critical to avoid consumption of toxic materials [64]. This makes us appreciate the importance of gustation in survival and quality of life.

Neurodegenerative disorders have underlying metabolic derangements [65, 66] associated with high sugar consumption [67]. Acute physical exercise also increases sweet intensity, sensitivity, and preference; however, chronic physical activity exerts opposite effects thereby reducing preferences for sweets [22]. Intensity, sensitivity, and preference for salty taste increase immediately after exercise but decreases later [21]. This shift may be explained by immediate calorie burning which is compensated by generating a preference for sweet taste to accommodate for the depleting glucose resources. The preference for salty taste immediately following exercise can be explained by the loss of body salts during perspiration in moderate- and high-intensity exercises. Yet the decline in preference and intensity of these tastes is evident later in the chronic physical activity state, reflecting the adaptation of the body after exercise. The implications of modulation of gustatory sense by physical activity are huge as it also modulates the preference for salty taste in obesity [19]. Metabolic diseases like obesity and diabetes pose a huge burden, both contributed by high-fat, high-processed, palatable diet. Hence, the burden of these metabolic disorders can be minimized by modulating taste preferences *via* moderate-intensity exercise.

2.5 Tactile sensation

Sense of touch is critical as it communicates toxic and mechanical insults received from the environment so that withdrawal from these insults could be done before they could cause great damage.

Loss of tactile sensation is evident in diabetic neuropathy [68] and neurodegenerative disorders [69, 70]. Loss of tactile sensations combined with peripheral vascular diseases worsens the condition and leads to gangrene [71, 72]. The goal of therapy in this case is to prolong independent and safe locomotion with reduces chances of physical deformity [73]. Among those therapeutic regimes, exercise is also included [73].

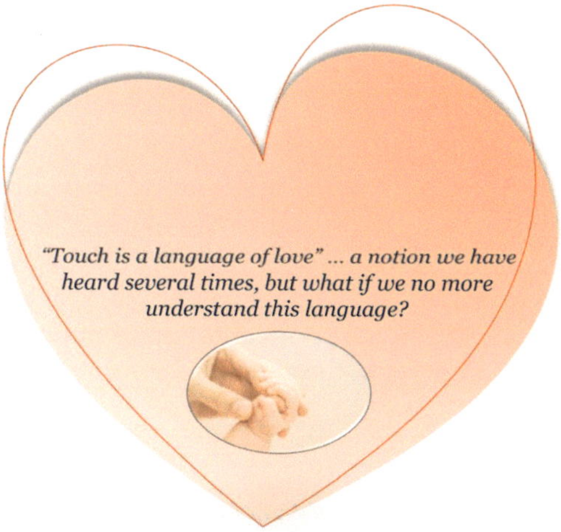

Moderate-intensity aerobic intervention for 8 weeks has shown tremendous effects in delaying progression of diabetic peripheral neuropathy [74] and improving nerve regeneration [75] with visible impact on structural modification, axonal phenotype, and release of neurotrophic factors. Moderate-intensity exercise acts by reducing myelin-associated glycoprotein (MAG) expression in the spinal cord [76]. In a rat model of sciatic nerve injury, 3–7 day training on voluntary wheel exercise improved neurite outgrowth, the extent of which was associated with the distance performed by them [77], an effect contributed by increasing expression of brain-derived neurotrophic factor and synapsin [78]. By promoting these growth factors, exercise interventions enhance cutaneous innervation in diabetic peripheral neuropathy [79].

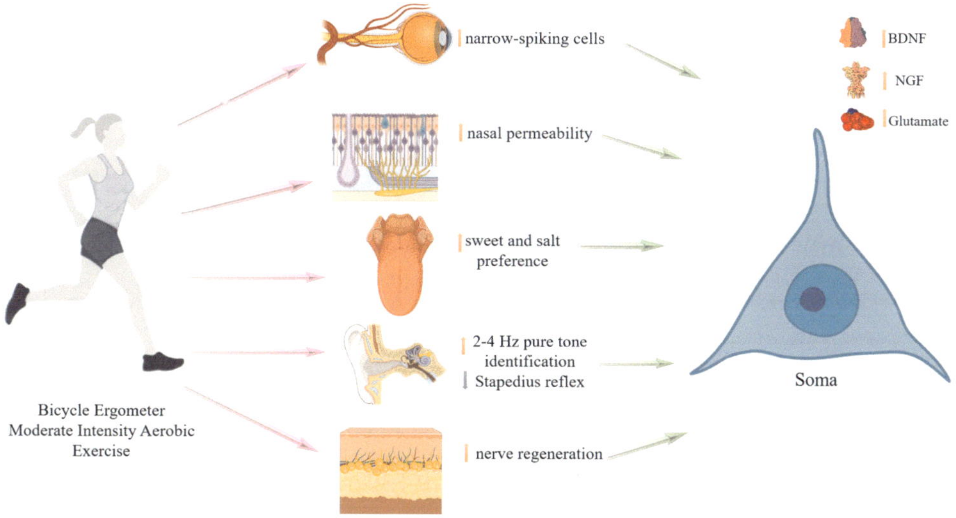

Figure 1.
Impact of exercise on perception via five senses. Moderate-intensity exercises and bicycle ergometer activate narrow-spiking cells in the visual system, increase nasal permeability, enhance preference for sweet and salty taste, improves pure tone identification, and facilitates nerve regeneration in the skin by the action of brain-derived neurotrophic factors (BDNF), nerve-growth factor (NGF), and glutamine. Figure developed using Biorender.

Consequently, motor rehabilitation improves tactile sensation following stroke [80], thereby reinforcing the role of physical activity in improving tactile sensations and minimizing prevalence of skin ulcerations (**Figure 1**).

3. Executive function

Executive functions involve high-level thinking skills mainly in the areas like working memory that also involves attention and cognitive flexibility reflected by the planning and decision-making and inhibition, which reflects self-control. Active lifestyle can enhance executive functions. Aerobic exercise, for example, improves cognitive functions [81, 82]. It is therefore critical to mention how physically active lifestyle modulates brain functions as discussed below:

3.1 Attention

Attention is broadly categorized into four main types: selective, sustained, alternating, and divided. Functional categorization of attention from attention network theory defines it in three components that are alerting, orientation, and control [83]. It is a critical feature especially in the contemporary world, loaded with information and offering more mentally challenging professions than physically challenging ones in the previous century. We now observe increasing prevalences of attention deficits from young children having ADHD [84, 85] to loss of attentive capacity in neurodegenerative disorders [86–88].

Many studies have highlighted the role of acetylcholine receptors, both muscarinic and nicotinic, in aiding attention [89–92]. In addition to acetylcholine, dopamine [92, 93], norepinephrine [94], and glutamate [95, 96] have also been implemented in aiding attention. However, it would be too naïve if we rely on assuming that only neurotransmitters play an important role in attention. We also realize that the brain relies on networking for executive functions like attention. Hence, it is also critical that we discuss attentional networks to observe the impact of exercise on the functioning of those areas. Diffusion weighted imaging has revealed the involvement of the pulvinar, superior colliculi, the head of caudate nuclei, and the brain stem in dorsal (DAN) and ventral attention networks (VAN) [97]. However, a previously well-described role of medial prefrontal, frontal, and parietal activation in attention has also been established [98–100]. While discussing the effects of exercise, we will now focus on both the neurotransmission and attention networks to identify the potential mechanisms of exercise in brain function.

Exercise enhances dopamine levels [101, 102] by activating tyrosine hydroxylase, yet reduced the increased striatal dopamine after cerebral infarction [103], thereby serving a protective function. Voluntary wheel running reduces norepinephrine levels in locus coeruleus (LC) and its target regions, during stress by enhancing galanin expression [104]. Since LC is responsible for fear conditioning and norepinephrine is the primary neurotransmitter in LC, reduction in its level may alleviate fear responses, thereby reducing increasing metabolic demand in the brain. Serotonin (5-hydroxytrytamine: 5-HT), also known as the "happy hormone," is also modulated by different type of exercises. For example, 4 weeks of moderate treadmill exercise reduced 5-HT levels in hippocampus and amygdala, without compromising its metabolism [105, 106], while 4 weeks of running wheel exercise improves 5-HT metabolite concentration in striatum [107].

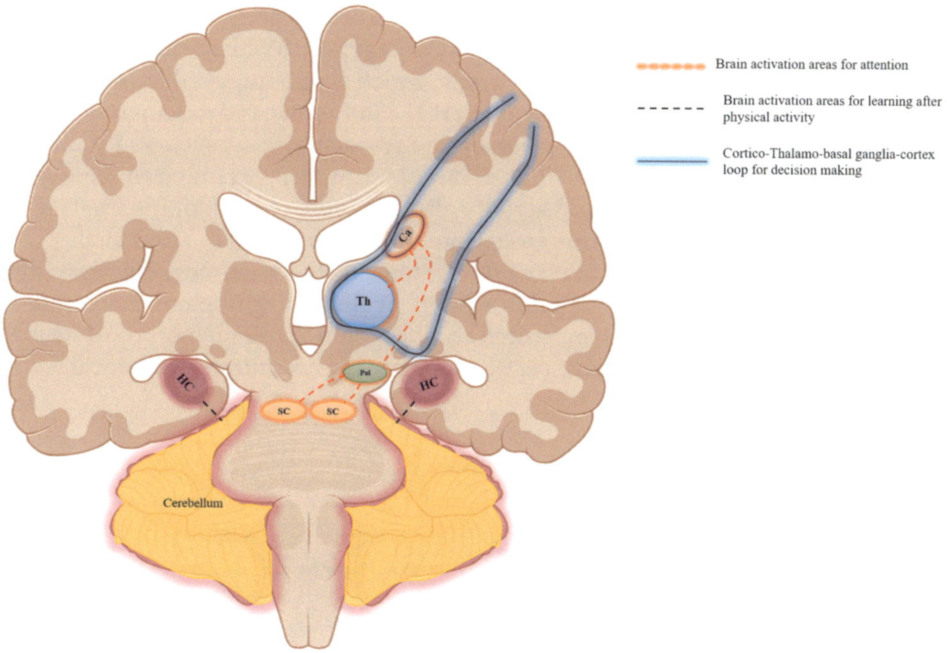

Figure 2.
Activation of executive function pathways by exercise. Red-dotted areas indicate brain circuitry for attention including superior colliculus (SC), pulvinar (Pu), caudate nucleus (Ca), and thalamus (Th), other than dorsal and ventral attention networks. Black-dotted lines indicate the brain areas involved in learning activation after exercise, including cerebellum and hippocampus (HC). Blue bold line indicates areas of decision making, which involves the activation of cortico-basal ganglia-thalamo-cortical loop. Figure created in Biorender.

Attention is modulated by the neurotransmitters discussed above where dopamine [108] plays a role in cortical maturation and specification required for attention. Selective attention requires focus, which in turn requires effort. The efforts required for the selective attention is modulated by the serotonin levels [109, 110]. Also, sustained attention is modulated by serotonin in the thalamus and caudate nucleus [111]. Hence, exercise influences response time in selective attention tasks [27]. Moreover, acute aerobic exercise also enhances selective attention in visual search tasks [28, 29]. Endurance exercises have shown remarkable effects on sustained attention [29]. Moderate-intensity exercise improves sustained attention as compared to low-intensity exercise [112]. Further delineation of moderate-intensity exercise with constant and variable-load revealed faster responses with preserved accuracy for variable loads in sustained attention tasks [112, 113]. There have been some evidences on the effect of aerobic exercise on alternating attention [114, 115] and divided attention [116]; however, further research is needed to enhance understanding on the effects of exercise on the other two types of attention (**Figure 2**).

3.2 Learning and memory

Memory can be broadly divided into short-term and long-term memory where short-term memory only works on synapses, long-term memory results in the activation of neurotransmitter signaling pathways that will in turn activate downstream signaling molecules such as cAMP, MAP kinases, and calcium calmodulin-dependent pathways [117].

Exercise-induced mitochondrial biogenesis involves the activation of $PGC1_{\alpha}$ *via* PPAR-$_{\gamma}$ [118], which is also evident in hippocampus [119]. We have also previously discussed that exercise enhances BDNF levels, which is also involved in increasing $PGC1_{\alpha}$ levels and mitochondrial biogenesis [119]. Glutamine and glutamate, the excitatory neurotransmitters are also enhanced after acute exhaustive endurance exercise [30] specially in the cerebellum and hippocampus, pertaining to increased oxygen demand. Similarly, physical activity also enhances the dopamine levels in adulthood [23]. Specifically high-intensity interval training (HIIT) also enhances dopamine signaling [120] in substance use disorder. Also, in neurodegenerative disorders intense exercise increase dopamine levels by increasing dopamine receptors and neuromelanin. Exercise also enhances acetylcholine/nestin phenotype of neurons, thereby enhancing spatial behavior [121]. These neurotransmitters are critical for learning and memory function.

> ....So let the light guide your way, yeah
> Hold every memory as you go
> And every road you take
> Will always lead you home, home ....
>
> At this point, how many of us can recall these lyrics from Wiz Khalifa's "see you again"?
>
> How many of us wonder if we do retain EVERY memory? If not, what helps us retain the ones we do?

Aerobic exercise increases anterior hippocampal volume [122] and improves spatial learning. One-year aerobic exercise is deemed sufficient for enhancing hippocampal volume even in late adulthood [31]. Both aerobic and resistance exercises enhance recognition memory by reducing acetylcholine esterase in amyloid beta-induced rat model of Alzheimer's disease [32, 33]. The process of memory formation involves encoding, storage, and retrieval. Even single-exercise workout improves memory encoding by enhancing dopamine transporters [34, 123]. Acute exercise enhances free-recall memory [35] by enhancing recall accuracy [124] for short-term recall [11]. Hence, physical activity demonstrates a positive effect on memory encoding and recall. The mechanisms underlying exercise-induced memory consolidation are scarce [11, 12] and need further studies to establish their interaction with memory.

3.3 Decision-making

If we look at the decision-making circuitry, it involves the cortico-basal ganglia-thalamo-cortical (CBGTC) loop [125]. The nucleus accumbens in this loop contains dopamine D1 or D2 receptor-expressing medium spiny neuron (D1-/D2-MSN) [125]. So far, we have discussed how dopamine levels increase after acute exercise [120]. However, a direct modulation of dopamine-related reward pathway especially in the mesolimbic system influences decision-making [126]. Dopamine is also involved in reinforcement learning, which in turn affects decision-making [127], especially effort-based decision-making. Aerobic exercise, *via* the reward processing pathway, influences risky decision making in young adults [128]. Decision-making can be defined as a goal-directed behavior, which involves the cortico-basal ganglia circuit [129].

DOI: http://dx.doi.org/10.5772/intechopen.1013187

In cortex, dopamine neuronal terminals primarily lie in the layers I and V-VI where they radiate efferent projections to corticothalamic and corticostriatal areas [130].

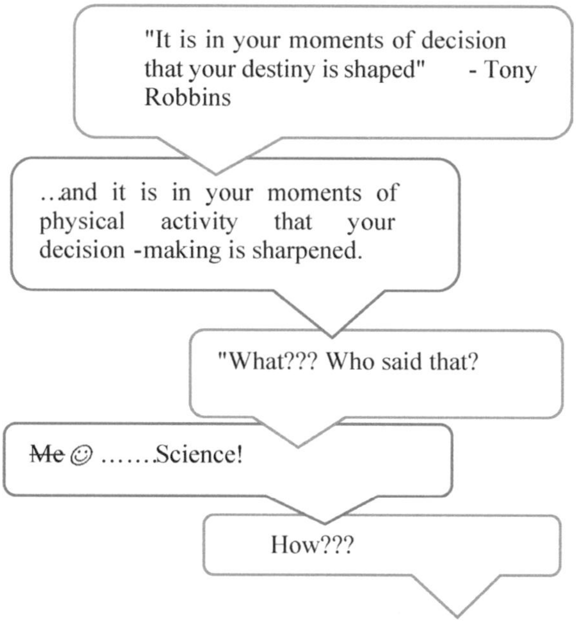

Exercise has the neuroprotective effects on the dopaminergic nigrostriatal pathway in Parkinson's disease [131]. Similar results have been observed in a sample of post-traumatic stress disorder (PTSD) women where model-based decision making was improved after moderate-intensity aerobic exercise [132]. However, in a sample of experienced vs. inexperienced soccer players, exercise only affected the speed of decision making instead of its accuracy [133]. Some decisions require desirability-feasibility trade-offs, which is also enhanced by regular leisure physical activity that makes the decisions less prone to dilution effects that refer to the mixing of relevant and irrelevant information, thereby making their judgments less extreme [14]. While these studies explain rational decision making, high-intensity exercise also improves intuitive decision making, required for demanding areas where quick decisions need to be made with good accuracy [134].

The influence of exercise on overall decision making is well established; however, the effect 0f exercise on different types of decision making is scarce. Further research on delineating this effect can enhance our understanding of modulation of different types of decision making by exercise.

3.4 Inhibition and self-control

Inhibition is an exciting idea in cognition, which advocates self-regulation and control in situations that otherwise may result in abrupt, violent, or reactive behaviors [135]. Inhibition or self-control is essential in maintaining a civilized society [135]. It is intriguing to learn that physical activity enhances self-control and inhibition [13, 20]. Specifically, unsupervised physical activity during breaktime in a sample of school children has shown strong association with inhibition control [18]. While the complete understanding of the brain circuitry for inhibitory responses is yet to be explored, tasks evaluating inhibitory control for alcohol use identified peak activations in the prefrontal regions specially inferior frontal gyrus, insula, middle frontal gyrus, supplementary motor area, precentral gyrus, and superior frontal gyrus of the right hemisphere, while insula and middle and superior frontal gyri activated in the left hemisphere [136]. Inhibition of intruding thoughts involves the fronto-temporal mnemonic pathway where dorsolateral prefrontal cortex (DLPFC) and ventrolateral prefrontal cortex (VLPFC) shift their modulation from M1 motor area to hippocampus after transitioning from action to thought stopping blocks [137]. It has been shown that motor control exercise can modify communication between default mode network and left-fronto parietal network, while moderate-intensity exercise increases medial prefrontal cortex activity [36]; however, no direct effect of exercise has been established in inhibition control circuitry as the realization of this circuitry is quite recent [137], which leaves an open arena of research on influence of exercise in inhibition and control as it could provide a valuable, cost-effective approach in improving symptoms in PTSD, addiction, and other disorders of inhibitory control.

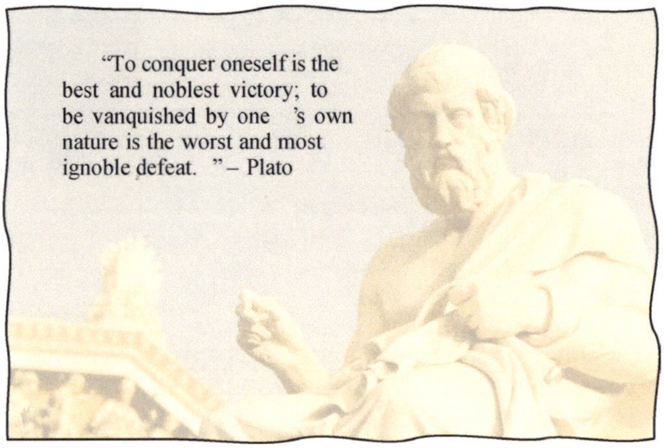

4. Language

Language requires rigorous word comprehension, especially in the semantic and pragmatic domains of language comprehension. Aerobic exercise enhances new word learning in school-aged children [138], while long-term follow-ups of exercise in children with learning disabilities also revealed improvement in reading [139]. Physical activity of other types improves new language learning in young-adults [9] and enhances language comprehension in monolingual older adults, an effect exerted by VO2 peak, yet it does not exert the same effects in the bilinguals for the second language [140]. The capacity of moderate-intensity long term exercise can thus be established for speech disorders. Speech disorders are currently rising and can potentially benefit greatly from moderate-intensity exercises. Hence, integration of moderate-intensity exercises can add value to the speech therapy protocols.

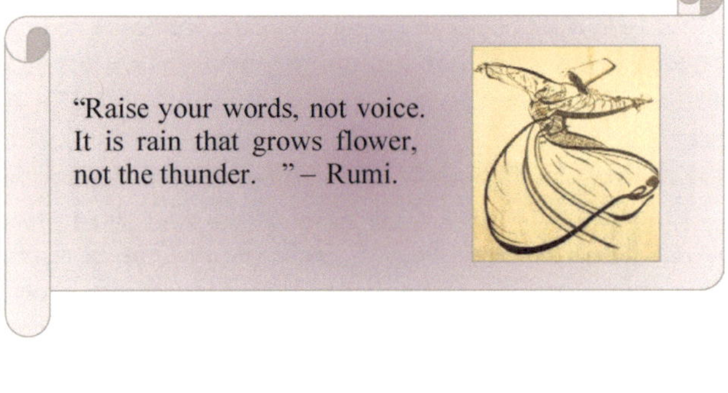

Exercise intervention has also been deemed effective in treating post-stroke aphasia [141]. High-intensity exercise has demonstrated improvement in word recall [142], word recognition, and spelling skills [143]. In healthy older adults, acute exercise enhances semantic memory activation specially in region including middle frontal, inferior temporal, middle temporal, and fusiform gyri [37], a network dedicated to semantic memory. Additional, bilateral activation in the hippocampus also occurs after acute exercise; however, the results from Ref. [37] were confined to correct trials only, hence it remained unknown how semantic disagreement could influence hippocampal activation after exercise.

Stroke-related aphasia significantly improves after exercise intervention, which may be attributed to improved blood flow and immune function in the brain, and further work is required to establish the effects of exercise in neurodegenerative disorders like aphasia associated with dementia, as it could be of great value in devising a rehabilitation regime for treating aphasia related to neurodegeneration.

5. Social and emotional cognition

Social cognition not only involves social intelligence but also emotional intelligence. Moderate-intensity exercise enhances social information processing and emotional understanding [144] and reduces social anxiety [145]. Physical activity also enhances social competence and improves interpersonal relationships among high-school students [7]. A body of research on the effects of physical activity supports its influence on emotional wellbeing [146], a skill necessary to navigate through relationships in different domains of life. Emotional reactivity is evident in depressive disorders that are effectively countered by even a single session of aerobic exercise [147]. Regular exercise provides beneficial effects in mitigating self-rated negative emotions in stress [148]. While this study posed limitation in ranking negative emotions because the emotions were self-rated, an 8-week intervention incorporating aerobic jogging also modulated the implicit emotion regulation ability [149]. Moreover, similar intervention in children also provided sufficient evidence for the regulation of negative emotions in children [24]. This effect is also evident in adults where physical activity not only improves resilience during stress but also enhance one's trait emotional intelligence [150, 151]. Improving social and emotional cognition can help in treating anxiety, personality, and affective disorders. Exercise improves symptoms in anxiety and elevates mood in affective disorders; however, further work can also explore the direct effects of exercise on personality disorders as they are difficult to treat with conventional therapies.

"The more socially intelligent you are, the happier and more robust and more enjoyable your relationships will be."
— Daniel Goleman

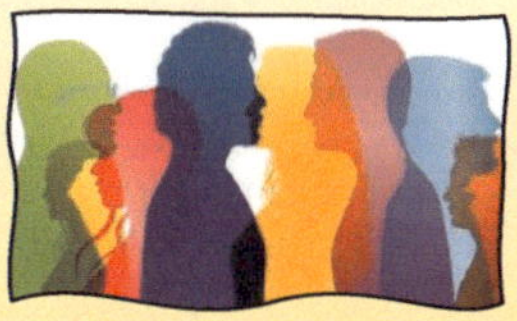

6. Interoception

Interoception is that ability to know oneself physiologically, a sense of internal body states. It includes the hunger pangs we get, midnight cravings, or racing hearts in the arousal states.

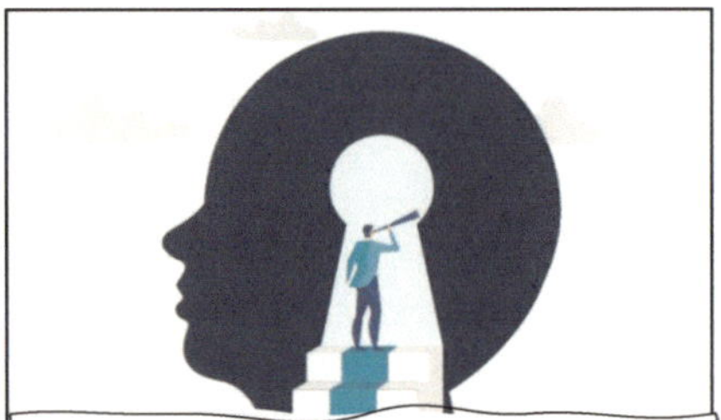

Mastering others is strength,
mastering yourself is true pow er -

Lao Tzu

The interoceptive system in the brain has recently been explored where afferent inputs from the visceral body are received in dorsal mid and posterior Insula [152]. The visceromotor prediction signals are sent to insular regions from the cingulate cortex while spanning some portion from the dorsal amygdala as amygdala has central nucleus which also facilitates visceromotor signals [152]. Primarily, vagus nerve supplies all body organs; hence, it also transmits signals from various organs along with small-diameter C and Aδ fibers [152]. Physical activity improves the interoceptive

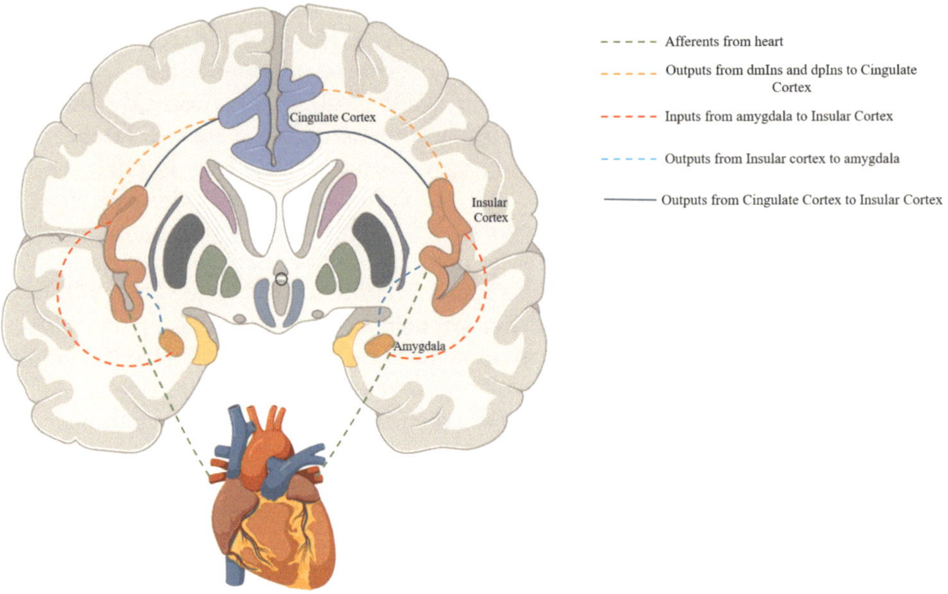

Figure 3.
Exercise-induced modulation of heart-brain communication. Brain receives visceral signals via *vagus and C and Aδ fibers in the dorsal medial (dmIns) and dorsal posterior insula (dpIns) (green-dotted lines), which send outputs to cingulate cortex (orange-dotted line) forming a bidirectional connection where it also receives input from cingulate cortex (blue bold line). Brain also forms a bidirectional connection with amygdala. Afferents from heart are received in amygdala which transmits signals to dmIns and dpIns (red-dotted line) which then send signals back to amygdala (blue dotted lines). Figure created in Biorender.*

accuracy in the heartbeat tracking task after 3 months of exercise [17]. While interoception requires attentional focus, physical activity enhances cardiac interoceptive accuracy independent of the attentional focus [136]. Physical activity exerts its effects *via* modulating the afferent inputs entering the interoceptive system [25]. The interoceptive system in the brain has recently been explored where afferent inputs from the visceral body are received in dorsal mid and posterior insula [152]. The visceromotor prediction signals are sent to insular regions from the cingulate cortex while spanning some portion from the dorsal amygdala as amygdala has central nucleus, which also facilitates visceromotor signals [152]. Cardiac awareness is more pronounced in self-regulated than externally prescribed exercises [153]. The positive effects of exercise are also evident in psychiatric disorders like depression [154] and substance use disorder [155]. Also, children with enhanced interoceptive sensitivity perform better at physical performance tasks [156], reflecting the bidirectional nature of this communication. Heartbeat-evoked potential is the neurophysiological index of interoception [157] and postulated to originate from intrinsic cardiac ganglia [158]. Lifelong aerobic exercise enhances the size of cardiac neurons and prevents them from age-related neurodegeneration [159], hence translating into the clinical effects of exercise on interoception [17, 160]. Improved interoception can contribute to early recognition of visceral disorders, especially cardiac disorders. Exercise, by modulating interoception, can influence visceral awareness. Clinical trials on different types of exercise can further enhance our understanding of the modulation of interoceptive pathways (**Figure 3**).

7. Conclusion

The importance of physical activity is evident and widely studied in metabolic disorders, rendering them as part of the therapeutic regime. Many well-known physical activity regimes have been devised into rehabilitation sciences to restore the body's physiological functions. However, the most accepted clinical effect of physical activity has been attributed to its protective effects in cardiovascular disorders as there is a general lack of prescription exercises in many other metabolic disorders. The brain, just like other organs, is also metabolically active. Metabolic disorders in the brain result in neurodegenerative diseases, which appear only later in life. The pathological mechanism initiates years earlier than the onset of symptoms, and hence, the right time to incorporate physical activity to enhance brain function is in the early ages. Physical activity not only enhances metabolism but also results in optimizing brain function. Several brain functions important for development, personality, and everyday working are influenced by physical activity. Moderate- to high-intensity exercises are proven to modulate molecular machinery in the five senses and central nervous system. It works by enhancing mainly excitatory neurotransmitters like dopamine and glutamate in the region of higher executive functions like attention, working memory, and inhibition. Interestingly, physical activity also enhances interoception, the internal state of awareness which is critical for survival. Physical activity also improves mood disorders and enhances one's ability for social cognition. Hence, physical activity must be incorporated into the therapeutic regimes targeting psychiatric and neurological conditions to improve the quality of life outcomes and ensure healthy aging.

Author details

Meha Fatima Aftab
Dow Institute of Medical Technology, Dow University of Health Sciences, Karachi, Pakistan

*Address all correspondence to: meha.fatima@duhs.edu.pk

References

[1] Harvey PD. Domains of cognition and their assessment. Dialogues in Clinical Neuroscience. 2019;**21**(3):227-237

[2] von Loeffelholz C, Birkenfeld AL. Non-Exercise Activity Thermogenesis in Human Energy Homeostasis. [Updated 2022 Nov 25]. In: Feingold KR, Adler RA, Ahmed SF, et al., editors. Endotext [Internet]. South Dartmouth (MA): MDText.com, Inc.; 2000-. Available from: https://www.ncbi.nlm.nih.gov/books/NBK279077/

[3] Westcott WL. Resistance training is medicine: Effects of strength training on health. Current Sports Medicine Reports. 2012;**11**(4):209-216

[4] Shepherd JT. Circulatory response to exercise in health. Circulation. 1987;**76**(6 Pt. 2):VI3-V10

[5] Delp MD et al. Exercise increases blood flow to locomotor, vestibular, cardiorespiratory and visual regions of the brain in miniature swine. The Journal of Physiology. 2001;**533**(Pt. 3):849-859

[6] Hellstrom G, Wahlgren NG. Physical exercise increases middle cerebral artery blood flow velocity. Neurosurgical Review. 1993;**16**(2):151-156

[7] Hu Y et al. Research on the mechanism of the impact of physical activity on negative emotions of middle school students, and the chain mediating role of social competence and interpersonal relationships. Frontiers in Psychology. 2025;**16**:1577987

[8] Neeper SA et al. Physical activity increases mRNA for brain-derived neurotrophic factor and nerve growth factor in rat brain. Brain Research. 1996; **726**(1–2):49-56

[9] Liu F et al. It takes biking to learn: Physical activity improves learning a second language. PLoS One. 2017;**12**(5): e0177624

[10] Maddock RJ et al. Acute modulation of cortical glutamate and GABA content by physical activity. The Journal of Neuroscience. 2016;**36**(8):2449-2457

[11] Marchant D et al. The effects of acute moderate and high intensity exercise on memory. Frontiers in Psychology. 2020;**11**:1716

[12] Jentsch VL, Wolf OT. Acute physical exercise promotes the consolidation of emotional material. Neurobiology of Learning and Memory. 2020;**173**:107252

[13] Li X et al. Effect of exercise on inhibitory control is dose-dependent for adolescents. Sports Medicine and Health Science. 2022;**4**(1):54-60

[14] Zimmermann L, Chakravarti A. Not just for your health alone: Regular exercisers' decision-making in unrelated domains. Journal of Experimental Psychology. Applied. 2022;**28**(2):379-398

[15] Fonseca MT et al. Effects of physical exercise in nasal volume. Brazilian Journal of Otorhinolaryngology. 2006; **72**(2):256-260

[16] Namiranian K et al. The association between parameters of physical activity and olfactory function-the importance of frequency and moderate intensity. Frontiers in Sports and Active Living. 2024;**6**:1394858

[17] Amaya Y et al. The effect of aerobic exercise on interoception and cognitive function in healthy university students: A non-randomized controlled trial. BMC Sports Science, Medicine and Rehabilitation. 2021;**13**(1):99

[18] Watson E, Burgess PW, Xu C, Boulton H, Habib SM, Metcalf I, et al.

Association between physical activity and inhibitory control in children. International Journal of Sport and Exercise Psychology. 2025;**23**(7):1256-1272. DOI: 10.1080/1612197X.2024.2393303

[19] Santos MMD et al. Taste sensitivity, food preferences, and physical activity pattern associated with nutritional status of adolescents. Journal of Sensory Studies. 2019;**34**(3):e12491

[20] Cheng L et al. Exploring the effects of long-term physical exercise on persistent and inhibitory self-control: Quasi-experimental research. Frontiers in Sports and Active Living. 2025;**7**: 1543481

[21] Gauthier AC, Dupont F, Mathieu ME. Association between physical activity and taste-the advantage of increased intensity for some but not all individuals. PLoS One. 2023;**18**(12): e0295173

[22] Gauthier AC et al. Effect of physical exercise on taste perceptions: A systematic review. Nutrients. 2020;**12**(9):1-24

[23] Marques A et al. Bidirectional association between physical activity and dopamine across adulthood-A systematic review. Brain Sciences. 2021;**11**(7):1-14

[24] Li J et al. Exercise intervention and improvement of negative emotions in children: A meta-analysis. BMC Pediatrics. 2023;**23**(1):411

[25] Wallman-Jones A et al. Physical activity and interoceptive processing: Theoretical considerations for future research. International Journal of Psychophysiology. 2021;**166**:38-49

[26] Harnish SM et al. Aerobic exercise as an adjuvant to aphasia therapy: Theory, preliminary findings, and future directions. Clinical Therapeutics. 2018; **40**(1):35-48 e6

[27] Coleman M, Offen K, Markant J. Exercise similarly facilitates men and women's selective attention task response times but differentially affects memory task performance. Frontiers in Psychology. 2018;**9**:1405

[28] Bullock T, Giesbrecht B. Acute exercise and aerobic fitness influence selective attention during visual search. Frontiers in Psychology. 2014;**5**:1290

[29] Ligeza TS et al. Acute aerobic exercise benefits allocation of neural resources related to selective attention. Scientific Reports. 2023;**13**(1): 8624

[30] Swiatkiewicz M et al. Increases in brain (1)H-MR glutamine and glutamate signals following acute exhaustive endurance exercise in the rat. Frontiers in Physiology. 2017;**8**:19

[31] Erickson KI et al. Exercise training increases size of hippocampus and improves memory. Proceedings of the National Academy of Sciences of the United States of America. 2011;**108**(7): 3017-3022

[32] Farzi MA et al. Exercise improves recognition memory and acetylcholinesterase activity in the beta amyloid-induced rat model of Alzheimer's disease. Annals of Neurosciences. 2019;**25**(3):121-125

[33] Loprinzi PD et al. Acute and chronic exercise effects on human memory: What we know and where to go from here. Journal of Clinical Medicine. 2021; **10**(21):1-16

[34] Chaire A, Becke A, Duzel E. Effects of physical exercise on working memory and attention-related neural

oscillations. Frontiers in Neuroscience. 2020;**14**:239

[35] Pesce C et al. Physical activity and mental performance in preadolescents: Effects of acute exercise on free-recall memory. Mental Health and Physical Activity. 2009;**2**(1):16-22

[36] Kimura D et al. Effects of different exercise intensities on prefrontal activity during a dual task. Scientific Reports. 2022;**12**(1):13008

[37] Won J et al. Semantic memory activation after acute exercise in healthy older adults. Journal of the International Neuropsychological Society. 2019;**25**(6): 557-568

[38] Niell CM, Stryker MP. Modulation of visual responses by behavioral state in mouse visual cortex. Neuron. 2010; **65**(4):472-479

[39] Fu Y et al. A cortical disinhibitory circuit for enhancing adult plasticity. eLife. 2015;**4**:e05558

[40] Maddock RJ et al. Vigorous exercise increases brain lactate and Glx (glutamate+glutamine): A dynamic 1H-MRS study. NeuroImage. 2011;**57**(4): 1324-1330

[41] Wang HF et al. Hearing impairment is associated with cognitive decline, brain atrophy and tau pathology. eBioMedicine. 2022;**86**:104336

[42] Cristell M, Hutchinson KM, Alessio HM. Effects of exercise training on hearing ability. Scandinavian Audiology. 1998;**27**(4):219-224

[43] Martinez-Amezcua P et al. The association between midlife leisure-time physical activity and hearing loss in late life in the atherosclerosis risk in communities study. The Journals of Gerontology. Series A, Biological Sciences and Medical Sciences. 2023; **78**(7):1292-1299

[44] Colletti V et al. Reduced active protection to the cochlea during physical exercise. Acta Oto-Laryngologica. 1991; **111**(2):234-239

[45] Assi S et al. Hearing loss and physical activity among older adults in the United States. The Journals of Gerontology. Series A, Biological Sciences and Medical Sciences. 2024;**79**(1):1-8

[46] Li L et al. Hearing loss and gait speed among older adults in the United States. Gait & Posture. 2013;**38**(1):25-29

[47] Chen DS et al. Association of hearing impairment with declines in physical functioning and the risk of disability in older adults. The Journals of Gerontology. Series A, Biological Sciences and Medical Sciences. 2015; **70**(5):654-661

[48] Cournoyer M, Gauthier AC, Maldera A, Maso FD, Mathieu ME. Effect of physical activity on olfaction acuity: A systematic review. Physiology & Behavior. Oct 2024;**284**:114648. DOI: 10.1016/j.physbeh.2024.114648

[49] Papazian EJ, Pinto JM. Olfactory loss and aging: Connections with health and well-being. Chemical Senses. 2021;**46**:1-13

[50] Gregori D et al. Understanding the influence of the snack definition on the association between snacking and obesity: A review. International Journal of Food Sciences and Nutrition. 2011; **62**(3):270-275

[51] Catamo E et al. Differences in taste and smell perception between type 2 diabetes mellitus patients and healthy

controls. Nutrition, Metabolism, and Cardiovascular Diseases. 2021;**31**(1): 193-200

[52] Sollai G, Crnjar R. Age-related olfactory decline is associated with levels of exercise and non-exercise physical activities. Frontiers in Aging Neuroscience. 2021;**13**:695115

[53] Marioni G et al. Nasal functional modifications after physical exercise: Olfactory threshold and peak nasal inspiratory flow. Rhinology. 2010;**48**(3): 277-280

[54] Zhang C, Li D, Wang X. Role of physical exercise type in olfactory deterioration in ageing. Rhinology. 2020; **58**(2):145-150

[55] Schubert CR et al. Odor detection thresholds in a population of older adults. Laryngoscope. 2017;**127**(6): 1257-1262

[56] Bonini M, Usmani OS. Let research leave you breathless, not physical exercise! ERJ Open Research. 2018;**4**(1):1-15

[57] Cicchella A, Stefanelli C, Massaro M. Upper respiratory tract infections in sport and the immune system response. A Review. Biology (Basel). 2021;**10**(5): 1-4

[58] Atias-Varon D, Heled Y. Strenuous and prolonged exercise and upper respiratory tract infection - treatment or threat? Harefuah. 2017;**156**(11): 730-734

[59] Kurowski M et al. Winter ambient training conditions are associated with increased bronchial hyperreactivity and with shifts in serum innate immunity proteins in young competitive speed skaters. Archives of Medical Science. 2018;**14**(1):60-68

[60] Lagunas-Rangel FA. G protein-coupled receptors that influence lifespan of human and animal models. Biogerontology. 2022;**23**(1):1-19

[61] Chubak J et al. Moderate-intensity exercise reduces the incidence of colds among postmenopausal women. The American Journal of Medicine. 2006; **119**(11):937-942.e5

[62] Sakai M et al. Gustatory dysfunction as an early symptom of semantic dementia. Dementia and Geriatric Cognitive Disorders Extra. 2017;**7**(3): 395-405

[63] Suto T et al. Disorders of "taste cognition" are associated with insular involvement in patients with Alzheimer's disease and vascular dementia: "memory of food is impaired in dementia and responsible for poor diet". International Psychogeriatrics. 2014;**26**(7): 1127-1138

[64] Perry E, Walton K, Lambert K. Prevalence of malnutrition in people with dementia in long-term care: A systematic review and meta-analysis. Nutrients. 2023;**15**(13):1-7

[65] De La Monte SM. Metabolic derangements mediate cognitive impairment and Alzheimer's disease: Role of peripheral insulin-resistance diseases. Panminerva Medica. 2012; **54**(3):171-178

[66] de la Monte SM. The full spectrum of Alzheimer's disease is rooted in metabolic derangements that drive type 3 diabetes. Advances in Experimental Medicine and Biology. 2019;**1128**:45-83

[67] Moreira PI. High-sugar diets, type 2 diabetes and Alzheimer's disease. Current Opinion in Clinical Nutrition and Metabolic Care. 2013;**16**(4): 440-445

[68] Norrsell U et al. Tactile directional sensibility and diabetic neuropathy. Muscle & Nerve. 2001;**24**(11): 1496-1502

[69] Loffler A et al. Reduced tactile sensitivity is associated with mild cognitive impairment. eBioMedicine. 2024;**99**:104896

[70] Kesayan T et al. Abnormal tactile pressure perception in Parkinson's disease. Journal of Clinical and Experimental Neuropsychology. 2015; **37**(8):808-815

[71] Dogiparthi SN et al. Cutaneous manifestations of diabetic peripheral neuropathy. Dermato-Endocrinology. 2017;**9**(1):e1395537

[72] Bodman MA, Dreyer MA, Varacallo MA. Diabetic peripheral neuropathy. In: StatPearls. Treasure Island (FL): Ineligible Companies; 2025

[73] Carter GT. Rehabilitation management of peripheral neuropathy. Seminars in Neurology. 2005;**25**(2): 229-237

[74] Dixit S, Maiya AG, Shastry BA. Effect of aerobic exercise on peripheral nerve functions of population with diabetic peripheral neuropathy in type 2 diabetes: A single blind, parallel group randomized controlled trial. Journal of Diabetes and its Complications. 2014; **28**(3):332-339

[75] Udina E et al. Effects of activity-dependent strategies on regeneration and plasticity after peripheral nerve injuries. Annals of Anatomy. 2011; **193**(4):347-353

[76] Ghiani CA et al. Exercise decreases myelin-associated glycoprotein expression in the spinal cord and positively modulates neuronal growth. Glia. 2007;**55**(9):966-975

[77] Lopes CDF et al. BDNF gene delivery mediated by neuron-targeted nanoparticles is neuroprotective in peripheral nerve injury. Biomaterials. 2017;**121**:83-96

[78] Gomez-Pinilla F et al. Voluntary exercise induces a BDNF-mediated mechanism that promotes neuroplasticity. Journal of Neurophysiology. 2002;**88**(5):2187-2195

[79] Kluding PM et al. The effect of exercise on neuropathic symptoms, nerve function, and cutaneous innervation in people with diabetic peripheral neuropathy. Journal of Diabetes and its Complications. 2012; **26**(5):424-429

[80] Borstad A et al. Tactile sensation improves following motor rehabilitation for chronic stroke: The VIGoROUS randomized controlled trial. Neurorehabilitation and Neural Repair. 2022;**36**(8):525-534

[81] Smith PJ et al. Aerobic exercise and neurocognitive performance: A meta-analytic review of randomized controlled trials. Psychosomatic Medicine. 2010;**72**(3):239-252

[82] Ahn J, Kim M. Effects of aerobic exercise on global cognitive function and sleep in older adults with mild cognitive impairment: A systematic review and meta-analysis. Geriatric Nursing. 2023; **51**:9-16

[83] Schindler H et al. Molecular signatures of attention networks. Human Brain Mapping. 2024;**45**(3):e26588

[84] Abdelnour E, Jansen MO, Gold JA. ADHD diagnostic trends: Increased recognition or overdiagnosis? Missouri Medicine. 2022;**119**(5):467-473

[85] Westman E et al. Increase in occurrence of attention deficit

hyperactivity disorder differs by age group and gender-Finnish Nationwide Register Study. Brain and Behavior: A Cognitive Neuroscience Perspective. 2025;**15**(1):e70253

[86] Malhotra PA. Impairments of attention in Alzheimer's disease. Current Opinion in Psychology. 2019;**29**:41-48

[87] Stam CJ et al. Disturbed frontal regulation of attention in Parkinson's disease. Brain. 1993;**116**(Pt. 5):1139-1158

[88] Bloxham CA, Dick DJ, Moore M. Reaction times and attention in Parkinson's disease. Journal of Neurology, Neurosurgery, and Psychiatry. 1987;**50**(9):1178-1183

[89] Chudasama Y et al. Cholinergic modulation of visual attention and working memory: Dissociable effects of basal forebrain 192-IgG-saporin lesions and intraprefrontal infusions of scopolamine. Learning & Memory. 2004;**11**(1):78-86

[90] Hahn B, Shoaib M, Stolerman IP. Involvement of the prefrontal cortex but not the dorsal hippocampus in the attention-enhancing effects of nicotine in rats. Psychopharmacology. 2003;**168**(3): 271-279

[91] Hahn B, Shoaib M, Stolerman IP. Selective nicotinic receptor antagonists: Effects on attention and nicotine-induced attentional enhancement. Psychopharmacology. 2011;**217**(1):75-82

[92] Bentley P, Husain M, Dolan RJ. Effects of cholinergic enhancement on visual stimulation, spatial attention, and spatial working memory. Neuron. 2004; **41**(6):969-982

[93] Granon S et al. Enhanced and impaired attentional performance after infusion of D1 dopaminergic receptor agents into rat prefrontal cortex. The Journal of Neuroscience. 2000;**20**(3): 1208-1215

[94] Bradshaw SE et al. Age-related changes in prefrontal norepinephrine transporter density: The basis for improved cognitive flexibility after low doses of atomoxetine in adolescent rats. Brain Research. 2016;**1641**(Pt. B):245-257

[95] Murphy ER, Dalley JW, Robbins TW. Local glutamate receptor antagonism in the rat prefrontal cortex disrupts response inhibition in a visuospatial attentional task. Psychopharmacology. 2005;**179**(1):99-107

[96] Stefani MR, Groth K, Moghaddam B. Glutamate receptors in the rat medial prefrontal cortex regulate set-shifting ability. Behavioral Neuroscience. 2003; **117**(4):728-737

[97] Alves PN et al. The subcortical and neurochemical organization of the ventral and dorsal attention networks. Communications Biology. 2022;**5**(1): 1343

[98] Rossi AF et al. The prefrontal cortex and the executive control of attention. Experimental Brain Research. 2009; **192**(3):489-497

[99] Bissonette GB, Powell EM, Roesch MR. Neural structures underlying set-shifting: Roles of medial prefrontal cortex and anterior cingulate cortex. Behavioural Brain Research. 2013;**250**:91-101

[100] Williams JM, Mohler EG, Givens B. The role of the medial prefrontal cortex in attention: Altering predictability of task difficulty. Psychobiology. 1999; **27**(4):462-469

[101] Sutoo D, Akiyama K. Regulation of brain function by exercise. Neurobiology of Disease. 2003;**13**(1):1-14

[102] Meeusen R, De Meirleir K. Exercise and brain neurotransmission. Sports Medicine. 1995;**20**(3):160-188

[103] Mizutani K et al. Effects of exercise after focal cerebral cortex infarction on basal ganglion. Neurological Sciences. 2013;**34**(6):861-867

[104] Sciolino NR, Holmes PV. Exercise offers anxiolytic potential: A role for stress and brain noradrenergic-galaninergic mechanisms. Neuroscience and Biobehavioral Reviews. 2012;**36**(9): 1965-1984

[105] Chen HI et al. Treadmill exercise enhances passive avoidance learning in rats: The role of down-regulated serotonin system in the limbic system. Neurobiology of Learning and Memory. 2008;**89**(4):489-496

[106] Chennaoui M et al. Effects of physical training on functional activity of 5-HT1B receptors in rat central nervous system: Role of 5-HT-moduline. Naunyn-Schmiedeberg's Archives of Pharmacology. 2000;**361**(6): 600-604

[107] Renoir T et al. Effect of enhanced voluntary physical exercise on brain levels of monoamines in Huntington disease mice. PLoS Currents. 2011;**3**: RRN1281

[108] Nieoullon A. Dopamine and the regulation of cognition and attention. Progress in Neurobiology. 2002;**67**(1): 53-83

[109] Enge S et al. On the role of serotonin and effort in voluntary attention: Evidence of genetic variation in N1 modulation. Behavioural Brain Research. 2011;**216**(1):122-128

[110] Lockhofen DEL, Mulert C. Neurochemistry of visual attention. Frontiers in Neuroscience. 2021;**15**: 643597

[111] Wingen M et al. Sustained attention and serotonin: A pharmaco-fMRI study. Human Psychopharmacology. 2008; **23**(3):221-230

[112] Radel R, Tempest GD, Brisswalter J. The long and winding road: Effects of exercise intensity and type upon sustained attention. Physiology & Behavior. 2018;**195**:82-89

[113] Ciria LF et al. The relationship between sustained attention and aerobic fitness in a group of young adults. PeerJ. 2017;**5**:e3831

[114] Shams A et al. Effect of cognitive rehabilitation combined with physical exercise on sustained, selective, and alternating attention in school-aged girls attention-deficit/hyperactivity disorder. Iranian Journal of Psychiatry and Clinical Psychology. 2021;**3**:276-287. DOI: 10.32598/ijpcp.27.3.3342.1

[115] Flores-Ferro E et al. Neuroeducación Física: Efectos Del Ejercicio Aeróbico En La Atención Alternante, Planificación Y Memoria Visuoconstructiva En Estudiantes Universitarios. Revista Ecuatoriana de Neurología. 2023;**32**:25-31

[116] Hall CD et al. Cognitive and motor mechanisms underlying older adults' ability to divide attention while walking. Physical Therapy. 2011;**91**(7): 1039-1050

[117] Johnston MV, Alemi L, Harum KH. Learning, memory, and transcription factors. Pediatric Research. 2003;**53**(3): 369-374

[118] Yan Z. Exercise, PGC-1alpha, and metabolic adaptation in skeletal muscle.

Applied Physiology, Nutrition, and Metabolism. 2009;**34**(3):424-427

[119] Cheng A et al. Involvement of PGC-1alpha in the formation and maintenance of neuronal dendritic spines. Nature Communications. 2012;**3**:1250

[120] Tyler J et al. High intensity interval training exercise increases dopamine D2 levels and modulates brain dopamine signaling. Frontiers in Public Health. 2023;**11**:1257629

[121] Hall JM, Savage LM. Exercise leads to the re-emergence of the cholinergic/nestin neuronal phenotype within the medial septum/diagonal band and subsequent rescue of both hippocampal ACh efflux and spatial behavior. Experimental Neurology. 2016;**278**:62-75

[122] Moser MB et al. Spatial learning with a minislab in the dorsal hippocampus. Proceedings of the National Academy of Sciences of the United States of America. 1995;**92**(21):9697-9701

[123] Blomstrand P, Engvall J. Effects of a single exercise workout on memory and learning functions in young adults—A systematic review. Translational Sports Medicine. 2021;**4**(1):115-127

[124] Ahmadi S. The Effect of Physical Activity on Recall Accuracy; Memorizing Vocabulary in a Second Language. Tilburg University: Tilburg; 2016. p. 25

[125] Macpherson T et al. Editorial: Circuit, molecular, and developmental mechanisms in decision-making behavior. Frontiers in Neuroscience. 2023;**17**:1192237

[126] Gorrell S, Shott ME, Frank GKW. Associations between aerobic exercise and dopamine-related reward-processing: Informing a model of human exercise engagement. Biological Psychology. 2022;**171**:108350

[127] Kurniawan IT, Guitart-Masip M, Dolan RJ. Dopamine and effort-based decision making. Frontiers in Neuroscience. 2011;**5**:81

[128] Ludyga S et al. Acute effects of aerobic exercise on risky decision making and reward processing in young adults. Psychophysiology. 2025;**62**(3):e70029

[129] Haber SN. The place of dopamine in the cortico-basal ganglia circuit. Neuroscience. 2014;**282**:248-257

[130] Gaspar P, Stepniewska I, Kaas JH. Topography and collateralization of the dopaminergic projections to motor and lateral prefrontal cortex in owl monkeys. The Journal of Comparative Neurology. 1992;**325**(1):1-21

[131] Hou L et al. Exercise-induced neuroprotection of the Nigrostriatal dopamine system in Parkinson's disease. Frontiers in Aging Neuroscience. 2017;**9**:358

[132] Crombie KM, Azar A, Botsford C, Heilicher M, Hiser J, Moughrabi N, et al. The influence of aerobic exercise on model-based decision making in women with posttraumatic stress disorder. Journal of Mood and Anxiety Disorders. Aug 2023;**2**:100015. DOI: 0.1016/j.xjmad.2023.100015. Epub 2023 Jul 27. Erratum in: J Mood Anxiety Disord. 2023 Dec 10;4:100035. DOI: 10.1016/j.xjmad.2023.100035

[133] Fontana FE et al. Influence of exercise intensity on the decision-making performance of experienced and inexperienced soccer players. Journal of Sport & Exercise Psychology. 2009;**31**(2):135-151

[134] Faisal A et al. Effect of three months high-intensity anaerobic treadmill-based exercise on intuitive decision-making capability: A prospective cohort study. Journal of Human Sport and Exercise. 2024;**19**(3): 815-826

[135] Baumeister RF. Self-regulation, ego depletion, and inhibition. Neuropsychologia. 2014;**65**:313-319

[136] Weafer J et al. Neural correlates of inhibitory control are associated with stimulant-like effects of alcohol. Neuropsychopharmacology. 2021;**46**(8): 1442-1450

[137] Anderson MC, Crespo-Garcia M, Subbulakshmi S. Brain mechanisms underlying the inhibitory control of thought. Nature Reviews Neuroscience. Jul 2025;**26**(7):415-437. DOI: 10.1038/s41583-025-00929-y. Epub 2025 May 16

[138] Pruitt M, Morini G. Examining the role of physical activity on word learning in school-aged children. Journal of Speech, Language, and Hearing Research. 2021;**64**(5):1712-1725

[139] Reynolds D, Nicolson RI. Follow-up of an exercise-based treatment for children with reading difficulties. Dyslexia. 2007;**13**(2):78-96

[140] Fernandes EG et al. Effects of increasing fitness through exercise training on language comprehension in monolingual and bilingual older adults: A randomized controlled trial. Neuropsychology, Development, and Cognition. Section B, Aging, Neuropsychology and Cognition. 2024: 1-33

[141] Mayer JF et al. Cognitive and linguistic benefits of aerobic exercise: A state-of-the-art systematic review of the stroke literature. Frontiers in Rehabilitation Sciences. 2021; **2**:785312

[142] Frith E, Sng E, Loprinzi PD. Randomized controlled trial evaluating the temporal effects of high-intensity exercise on learning, short-term and long-term memory, and prospective memory. The European Journal of Neuroscience. 2017;**46**(10):2557-2564

[143] Jensen OE et al. The effects of physical activity interventions on prereading, early word recognition and spelling development in children: A systematic review and meta-analysis. Educational Research Review. 2025;**47**: 100668

[144] Zhang A-D, Peng-Fei Z, Sun H-Q. The effect of exercise on social cognitive function in adolescents: The mechanism of emotion. Cogent Education. 2025; **12**(1):2440178

[145] Wu J et al. The impact of physical exercise on adolescent social anxiety: The serial mediating effects of sports self-efficacy and expressive suppression. BMC Sports Science, Medicine and Rehabilitation. 2025;**17**(1):57

[146] Li J et al. The effects of physical activity on positive emotions in children and adolescents: A systematic review and meta-analysis. International Journal of Environmental Research and Public Health. 2022;**19**(21):1-18

[147] Ligeza TS et al. The effects of a single aerobic exercise session on mood and neural emotional reactivity in depressed and healthy young adults: A late positive potential study. Psychophysiology. 2023;**60**(1):e14137

[148] Childs E, de Wit H. Regular exercise is associated with emotional resilience to acute stress in healthy adults. Frontiers in Physiology. 2014;**5**:161

[149] Zhang Y et al. How does exercise improve implicit emotion regulation ability: Preliminary evidence of mind-body exercise intervention combined with aerobic jogging and mindfulness-based yoga. Frontiers in Psychology. 2019;**10**:1888

[150] Wu R et al. Effects of physical activity on regulatory emotional self-efficacy, resilience, and emotional intelligence of nurses during the COVID-19 pandemic. Frontiers in Psychology. 2022;**13**:1059786

[151] Solanki D, Lane AM. Relationships between exercise as a mood regulation strategy and trait emotional intelligence. Asian Journal of Sports Medicine. 2010; **1**(4):195-200

[152] Kleckner IR et al. Evidence for a large-scale brain system supporting allostasis and interoception in humans. Nature Human Behaviour. 2017:1

[153] Butterworth JB et al. Having the heart to exercise control: Cardiac interoception influences self-paced exercise regulation. European Journal of Sport Science. 2025;**25**(3):e12263

[154] Sun Q et al. The mediating role of interoceptive sensitivity in the relationship between physical activity and depression symptoms in college students. Behavioral Sciences (Basel). 2024;**14**(7):1-11

[155] Brevers D et al. Physical exercise to redynamize interoception in substance use disorders. Current Neuropharmacology. 2024;**22**(6): 1047-1063

[156] Georgiou E et al. Interaction of physical activity and interoception in children. Frontiers in Psychology. 2015; **6**:502

[157] Tanaka Y et al. Heartbeat evoked potentials reflect interoceptive awareness during an emotional situation. Scientific Reports. 2025;**15**(1):8072

[158] Aftab MF. Intrinsic cardiac neurons as the consulate general of the brain in the heart: A review. Brain & Heart. 2024; **2**(2):1-10

[159] Gama EF et al. Exercise changes the size of cardiac neurons and protects them from age-related neurodegeneration. Annals of Anatomy. 2010;**192**(1):52-57

[160] Zarza-Rebollo JA, Sanabria D, Perakakis P. Can Increased Interoception Explain Exercise-Induced Benefits on Brain Function and Cognitive Performance?. PsyArXiv. 10 Apr 2019. DOI: 10.31234/osf.io/vghy7